The
Roper–Logan–Tierney
Model in Action

The Roper–Logan–Tierney Model in Action
C. NEWTON

Peplau's Model in Action
H. SIMPSON

Orem's Model in Action
S. CAVANAGH

Further models in preparation

Neumann's Model in Action
Riehl's Model in Action

The Roper–Logan–Tierney Model in Action

CHARLEEN NEWTON

RGN, Dip.Nursing (Lond.)
Research & Development Department,
Royal Hampshire County Hospital,
Winchester

Series Editor
BOB PRICE

BA, M.Sc., SRN, Cert.Ed.(Education)
Army Medical Services School of Nursing,
Woolwich

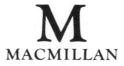

MACMILLAN

First published 1991 by
THE MACMILLAN PRESS LTD
Houndmills, Basingstoke, Hampshire RG21 2XS
and London
Companies and representatives
throughout the world

Designed by Claire Brodmann

ISBN 0–333–52134–X

A catalogue record for this book is available
from the British Library.

Printed in Hong Kong

Reprinted 1992 (twice), 1993

CONTENTS

The nursing profession has become increasingly familiar with the idea of nursing models, and has, at least in part, accepted them as a means to enhance nursing care. Such models have frequently emanated from the United States of America and have, quite naturally, been framed within the idiom and culture of American nurses. The Roper–Logan–Tierney model of nursing care provides a useful exception to this rule, and for many will be a framework of care that at once seems practical, approachable and functional.

The work of Roper, Logan and Tierney is widely known, but perhaps not fully understood within their native United Kingdom. British nurses are often tempted to select the 'activities of living' component of this model and to use this as a short checklist for care-giving, ignoring the model's other dimensions. This is a surprising mistake, given that this model is widely taught in Colleges of Nursing and espoused as a model of care for wards, departments and, sometimes, whole institutions. It is particularly apt, then, that Charleen Newton's refreshing look at this British model of nursing should be one of the first volumes in the *Nursing Models in Action* series.

Such a review is important for four very good reasons. First, and most generally, the profession has reached a point when all models of care are receiving critical attention. The early criticism of the medical model was well founded, but now, as the profession grows, we realise that we cannot rest on our own laurels, but must examine that which replaces the medical model. Nurses are asking the pertinent question, does this model of care enhance my practice, the way I care for a patient? If so, how does it do so and does this benefit hold good with all clients in every situation?

Charleen Newton's review is also important because many nurses will already be partially utilising this model of care, and may believe, perhaps erroneously, that they have grasped all its component parts and evaluated it fairly. In my experience this is often not the case. Activities of living are understood to the extent of compiling a check-list, but perhaps little more. The model is then evaluated, compared with others and found wanting, because the overlooked elements have not been given due attention. In this text the reader will enjoy a much fuller exploration of Roper, Logan and Tierney's work.

Thirdly, if this model is to be employed in college curricula, it is essential that it be reviewed, and applied to practical situations, by a nurse who is involved in the improved application of theory to practice. This author is ideally suited to this role, impartially examining the strengths and weaknesses of theory as she explores the best way to plan care in her own hospital setting. Fresh, research-related care studies are a feature of this text, and should prove invaluable to students and teachers of nursing alike.

Lastly, no model remains constant, and it will be clear from the following chapters that this one is no exception. It has developed and grown with the ongoing work of its authors and of those nurses who have sought to use this model of care. It is now appropriate to take stock of such change and – for nurses who seek to understand nursing theory – to put such work in the context of nursing culture and the current climate. The evaluation section of this text suits this purpose admirably, and will prove a welcome aid to those nurses studying at diploma, undergraduate or postgraduate level.

Reading through some of the texts on nursing models, you may be surprised to find the Roper–Logan–Tierney model unreferenced. Conversely, you may not be surprised at all, believing that this model doesn't quite fulfil the criteria of a classic nursing model. Either way, I suggest it's time to look again at all such beliefs and positions; an activity that is facilitated by this very practical book.

Bob Price

Certain conventions have been observed in the writing of this book. First, a person receiving nursing care is usually referred to as a 'patient', but in some contexts as a 'client'; the terms are often interchangeable and their use tends to be dictated by local practice. Secondly, although people in the book are introduced with their full names and titles they are usually referred to thereafter by their first name only – this reflects the trust established in effective nurse–patient relationships; each patient is understood to have consented to this use of his or her name. Thirdly, unless the context requires otherwise the nurse is referred to as 'she' and the patient as 'he'. These conventions are solely for reasons of simplicity, clarity and style.

ACKNOWLEDGEMENTS

I should like to thank my colleagues in the Research and Development Department at the Royal Hampshire County Hospital for their support and interest; the librarian and staff in the postgraduate medical centre at the Hospital for all their help; my supervisor at Southampton University for his encouragement and also patience in waiting for me to produce my thesis; Bob Price, the series editor, for his advice and inspiration; Andrew Nash, the copy-editor, for his help and patience; and finally my husband and family for spurring me on. I would also, of course, like to acknowledge the work of Roper, Logan and Tierney, which is the cornerstone of this book.

Charleen Newton

PART I

The Roper–Logan–Tierney model today

CHAPTER ONE

Models of nursing: a starting point

Oh, leave the jargons, and go your way straight to . . . work, in simplicity and singleness of heart.

(Nightingale 1859)

When Florence Nightingale wrote these words in 1859 it was to exhort nurses to give their best to the work they had chosen, despite the current jargons concerning rights of women. Today the word 'jargon' appears to have taken on a somewhat different meaning and is commonly understood as referring to a way of speaking, using words or terms peculiar to a particular group or profession. A first glance at nursing models may seem to reveal an overabundance of such jargon, and we as today's nurses are being exhorted to give our best to our chosen work by using a particular model of nursing in our area of practice. The model to be discussed in this book was designed by and for British nurses, so for them the problem of unfamiliar terms is minimal. One aim of this chapter, however, is to help nurses who may be unfamiliar with nursing models to negotiate a way safely through the common terminology of models, to emerge unscathed and eager to continue. The chapter will look at the development of nursing models in general and at the Roper–Logan–Tierney model in particular; it will discuss what is meant by the term 'nursing model'; it will examine the way nursing models are constructed; and it will explain the terms used to describe them. Finally we shall think about some of the reasons why nursing models are used.

IN THE BEGINNING

Before describing models of nursing in any detail, their development must be considered as part of the whole development of nursing and of the role of women in society. In the Western world, nursing became an occupation concerned with the sick during the evolution of scientific knowledge in the Renaissance period. At this time it was largely carried out by religious communities, who devoted their whole lives to devotion and caring. Later, in the nineteenth century, a new breed of predominantly male, university-educated doctors emerged, emphasising medicine's scientific knowledge base; as a result, the core of unqualified women carers, healers and midwives declined in status. The low status was not helped by the increase in the unscrupulous type of nurse, personified by Dickens' portrayal in *Martin Chuzzlewit* of Mrs Gamp.

It was in this climate that Florence Nightingale introduced the idea of nursing as a profession, through her quest to develop knowledge specific to nursing. She asserted that it was by nurses' observation and experience that such knowledge would be gained. Meleis (1985) identifies Nightingale's contribution to the evolution of the nursing model from the medical model as the first of four stages in the search to clarify the meaning of nursing and to establish a professional identity. This first stage, *practice*, reflected a need for practical care.

Nightingale, like other social reformers of the time, was concerned with the prevalence of sickness and industrial injury among the poor, and made nursing a respectable occupation by determinedly representing it as a role submissive to that of medicine, one of carrying out the more basic care required as an adjunct to the curative role of the doctor (Hagell 1989), a role congruent with the role of women at that time – caring, dutiful, altruistic, and subservient to men. Nightingale had a mental image of nursing as assisting the reparative process of the sick and maintaining the health of the well. Although her ideas were mainly related to the immediate environment of the patients, the holistic approach of her writing about nursing may be seen as a forerunner of the theoretical nursing models of today (Nightingale 1859).

It was to be nearly a hundred years before nurses started thinking seriously about the further development of nursing knowledge and theory, although during these years training for nurses had become mandatory. In the 1950s – the stage defined by Meleis as the *education and administration* stage – nursing skills and management were examined and efforts were made to begin to base them on scientific and theoretical foundations (Schrock 1981). Another major change of thinking at this time concerned the change from task-orientated to patient-centred nursing care (Abdellah *et al.* 1960). At the same time Orlando (1961) developed and introduced the 'nursing process', because of needs for curricular changes in education. The nursing process was formulated in order to provide a professional and disciplined framework for nursing practice, replacing the personal, intuitive approach (Meleis 1985). Chin and Jacobs (1983) describe the nursing process as a problem-solving process which provides a framework in which nurses can look at nursing as a deliberate, thoughtful and self-correcting activity. It was introduced to encourage nurses to reconsider critically the use of the medical model and to assist in attempts to redefine nursing. The General Nursing Council formally adopted the nursing process as a framework for patient care in 1977 (Faulkner 1985).

The next stage of development, identified by Meleis as the *research* stage, was a result of degree programmes for nurses in America in the 1960s and 70s, which encouraged nurses to publish their own ideas and demonstrate a commitment to the idea that nursing needed systematic enquiry in addition to medical knowledge. Nurses began to question the medical model – based on the biophysical sciences – in which man is seen as a biological being whose integrity is disturbed by disease, and in which the goal is to cure the disease by medical intervention. It was during this period that Nancy Roper was examining the learning experience of student nurses as part of a research study in Edinburgh, a study which resulted in the proposal of her model of nursing. Development of nursing models and theory – which expressed explicit individual beliefs about the concepts of the nursing role, the patient, the environment and health – grew out of this quest for new professional knowledge and status, a stage identified by Meleis as the stage of *theory*.

The search for professional identity through the years has been influenced by society's expectations for women and, as the majority of nurses are women, for nursing itself. Nurses have been seen as dependent on other disciplines for decision-making and have been valued only in relation to their observable activity, or 'busyness'. The development of nursing models is helping to establish nurses as thinkers as well, with a unique body of professional knowledge, while the application of a nursing model in practice not only provides a logical basis for patient care but also continues to add to that body of knowledge through experience and observation.

THE DEVELOPMENT OF THE ROPER–LOGAN–TIERNEY MODEL

The Roper–Logan–Tierney model of nursing was originally conceived and constructed by Nancy Roper in 1976 as part of a research study into nurse education, looking specifically at the clinical experience of learner nurses. The aim was to develop a conceptual framework reflecting the 'image' or 'idea' of nursing in order to consolidate the experience of learners in focusing on the patient as a whole, as an alternative to the fragmented medical approach of focusing on the disease.

In the thirty years preceding the study, the image of bedside nursing had predominated: before the introduction of early ambulation to prevent complications of bed rest, and before the improvement in pharmacology in the 1950s, many clinical conditions required long periods of bed rest. The nursing care at this time, designed to help patients carry out their usual daily living activities, took place at the bedside. However the term 'basic nursing' was used in the Nuffield report of 1953 to include all those activities of daily living for which the patient required nursing help. Roper's study looked at five of these activities – washing, mouth cleaning, dressing/undressing, eliminating, and feeding – and demonstrated that nursing decisions were used to assess the patients' abilities in these activities in order to determine their need for nursing care. She also established that it was the nurses' clinical judgement, based on individual patient needs, that identified the patients who required care to prevent the complications of bed rest. She recommended that the image of nursing should make explicit the common nursing requirements of all patients, despite their medical labels, and that learning objectives should be related to activities of daily living rather than clinical speciality (Roper 1976).

Further work by Roper, Logan and Tierney resulted in publication in 1980 of the first British model: *The Elements of Nursing* was written because of their belief that:

> The complexity and specialisation of nursing today makes it more necessary than ever for the elements of nursing to be identified and understood.
> (Roper *et al.* 1980)

In *Learning to Use the Process of Nursing*, published in 1981, they demonstrated the use of their model within the nursing-process framework, while in *Using a Model for Nursing* (1983) the model was applied to clinical situations by practising nurses.

WHAT IS A NURSING MODEL?

What do we understand by a nursing model? It might be helpful to consider what we understand by the term 'model' itself. Many examples will spring readily to mind – model toys such as trains and cars for imaginative play, or prototypes of complicated structures to be tested before production begins; each is a simulation, representing the real thing in manageable proportions. 'Model' may also be used to mean an ideal, an example, an image; or, with slightly different connotations, a pattern, a rule of thumb. Or in the words of Hazzard and Kergin (1971) a model is:

> a symbolic depiction in logical terms of an idealised, relatively simple situation showing the structure of the original system.

So a nursing model may be described as a mental, or conceptual, image of the ideal, of what nursing *should* be like, an image that provides direction, or a pattern, to achieve the model's goal. It is a representation of the reality of nursing in ideal terms.

Johnson (1975) defines a nursing model as:

> a systematically constructed, scientifically based and logically related set of concepts, which identify the essential components of nursing practice together with the theoretical base for these concepts and the values required in their use by the practitioner.
>
> (Riehl and Roy 1980)

There sometimes appears to be some confusion regarding the difference between the *nursing process* and a *nursing model*, and a definition proposed by Walsh (1989) puts this clearly in perspective using wonderfully simple terms:

> A model tells us what the nursing care should be like, the nursing process describes how it should be organised.

This demonstrates that the two must be used in harness – a principle that will provide the foundation for the description and application of the model in this book.

CONSTRUCTING A NURSING MODEL

It may be useful to base discussion of the construction of a nursing model on some of the terms used above in the definition given by Johnson.

The last phrase in the definition, 'values required ... by the practitioner', tells us that the beliefs and values (philosophy) underlying the model must be made explicit, not merely for theoretical reasons, but in order for the nurse to provide the required care. Each one of us holds beliefs and values about many subjects – our religion, our lifestyle, our political stance, our morality, ecology, child-rearing, learning: whatever we consider important in our lives. When we talk about any of these areas, we understand what we mean by the terms we use, but each word represents a huge array of abstract ideas, collectively called a *concept*. A dictionary definition of the word 'concept' includes words such as 'notion' and 'idea'; the thesaurus provides alternatives such as 'image', 'perception' or 'impression'. Chin and Jacobs (1983) define a concept as 'a complex mental formulation ... derived from individual perception and experience.' Torres (1985) quotes the above definition, among others, but asserts that nursing has used the term 'concept' for over fifty years without defining it. By the very nature of a concept – its being derived from individual experience – the image created may be different for each person and may generate endless ideas and interpretations.

As nurses, we hold beliefs about what we consider to be important in nursing, such as the quality of life, or health and illness, or our role as nurses, or the environment, and these are some of the concepts that identify the essential elements of nursing about which any nursing model must make an explicit statement of clarification. The major concepts discussed in this book are based on what Flaskerud and Halloran (1980) describe as four phenomena related to nursing:

- the nature of the individual (or patient/client);
- the nature of health and illness;
- the role of the nurse in health and illness;
- the environment.

These will also be discussed in the critique in Part III.

Johnson's definition also tells us that these concepts must be put together systematically and related to one another logically, and the next chapter will demonstrate how this is done in relation to the Roper–Logan–Tierney model.

The definition further states that there must be a theoretical base for the concepts. It is common to use the word 'theoretical' as opposite to 'practical', as though the two can never meet; it has connotations of academia, sometimes giving rise to the allegation that good practical nurses do not need to know a lot of theory, or that academic nurses are no good in practice. But consider some common practical activities, such as driving, cooking, DIY, or taking part in (or even watching) sports: they are all based on theory and to carry them out some of this theory has to be understood. Theory helps to describe, explain, predict and control practical events in real life: it has organisation and pattern, and it always serves some purpose (Chin and Jacobs 1983). It provides a structure to look at these events and to organise our understanding. Nursing theory provides the rationale for our nursing actions and helps to establish professional status.

It is possible to distinguish between the fundamental types of nursing model according to their theoretical foundations. Systems, development and interaction theories are the three main themes outlined by Riehl and Roy (1980), while Torres (1985) has in addition identified 'needs theory' as a major theme. Botha argues that no single theory should be seen as the exclusive approach of any model, but rather as a reflection of the major emphasis of the model (Botha 1989). With this in mind, a brief explanation of the distinctive characteristics of each of the theories mentioned above may help to identify and clarify the theoretical emphasis of the Roper–Logan–Tierney model.

Systems models

The human body is a system made up of several interrelated subsystems, and systems models focus on these physiological systems in addition to the psychological and social systems within the person as a whole. The key points of this theory are:

- All parts of a system interact with each other and have a common goal.
- Systems have a boundary which can be defined (skin).
- Systems strive to be in a state of equilibrium (homeostasis).
- Systems may be affected by stress, strain, tension and conflict.
- A system has feedback allowing change to maintain equilibrium.

Systems models make the assumption that nursing is required when the parts of the human system are not interacting effectively, or when stress occurs to disturb the equilibrium.

Development models

Development models concentrate on human development and assert that nursing care is required when the process of development is affected by illness or accident. The key points of this theory are these:

- The focus is on growth and directional change, usually with an increase in value at every stage of change.
- There must be identifiable stages of progression which can be differentiated from each other.
- There must be a specific form of progression, such as linear, with no reverting to previous stages, or spiral, where the same stages occur but at a higher developmental level.
- There must be some stimulus which produces the change: natural forces such as human growth or outside stimuli such as illness, social or educational factors.

(Adapted from Chin 1980)

Interaction models

Interaction models centre on the interaction between nurse and patient or client, and assume that interaction is meaningful, leading to adaptation of roles or behaviour. Interaction theory makes the following assumptions:

- Man's behaviour can be stimulated by interaction with others.
- Man can convey meanings and values by communication.
- Man can learn from communication with others.
- Thinking is a symbolic process, a rehearsal for future behaviour.

These models assert that nursing is required when a person cannot adopt a role that supports or sustains health (Rose 1980).

Needs theory

Needs theories argue that the ability of humans to survive is dependent on the extent to which their needs are met. The needs may be ordered hierarchically, as in a developmental needs theory: some needs are seen as having greater priority than others, as in Maslow's hierarchy of human needs, in which basic physiological needs take precedence over psychosocial needs (Torres 1985).

The extent to which the Roper–Logan–Tierney model reflects aspects of theory will be discussed in the next chapter.

WHY DO WE NEED NURSING MODELS?

Everyone would agree that nurses need to know what they are doing, and need to be able to explain why they are doing it. We would also agree that there needs to be consistency and continuity in the care given to a patient. A nursing model has already been described as a mental picture of nursing, and each nurse already has her own mental picture (even if it is never expressed in words), which may be different from that of every other nurse on the ward. It may, for example, be a picture of technological care, or of the medical/paternal picture of care, or an image of encouraging the patient to share in the responsibility for his own health. A specific nursing model, used by all the nurses, helps to ensure that all the nurses have the same 'picture', the same goal of nursing, the same knowledge to carry out the care. It ensures continuity and consistency, and the theoretical base provides a scientific rationale for care which increases nursing autonomy and control. It provides 'a common foundation of knowledge and thought processes on which to practice' (Chin and Jacobs 1983).

SUMMARY

This chapter has considered the development of nursing models as related to the development of nursing in the wider context of social and scientific change in Europe, America and Britain. Observations based on changes in British nursing care in the 1930s, 40s and 50s contributed to the construction of the model of nursing by Nancy Roper, who sought to develop a framework to help learner nurses focus on the patient as a person, rather than as a collection of clinical conditions.

Some of the terms commonly used when discussing nursing models have been defined in this chapter and may be summarised as follows:

Nursing model

A nursing model is a collection of mental images of what nursing should be like, which provides structure and direction to achieve its goal.

Concept

A concept is a complex mental picture or image, derived from individual experience. The key concepts which should be clear in any nursing model are:

- the nature of health;
- the nature of the individual receiving the care;
- the role of the nurse giving the care.

Theory

A theory is a scientifically acceptable, general principle which governs practice, or is proposed to explain observed facts.

(Riehl and Roy 1980)

The four theoretical foundations reflected most in nursing models are systems, development, interaction and needs theories. These theories form the base for the major emphasis of any model. Although some nursing models are described according to their theory base (as are Riehl's interaction model, Peplau's development model and Johnson's behavioural systems model), the Roper–Logan–Tierney model is commonly known as the 'Activities of Living model', not implying one major theoretical orientation but, as will be seen as the model is described, reflecting aspects of several.

CHAPTER TWO

The model of nursing and the nursing process

In this chapter and the next, the Roper–Logan–Tierney model of nursing is described in detail, including the original development, the key concepts of its philosophy, the five components of the model, the extent to which it reflects a theoretical base, and the way in which it may be put into practice within the framework of the nursing process.

The key concepts about which any model expresses its beliefs and values were identified in Chapter 1 as:

* the nature of the individual;
* the nature of health and illness;
* the role of nursing in health and illness;
* the nature of the environment.

These will be clarified and expanded in this chapter.

EARLY DEVELOPMENT

In 1976, when Nancy Roper first developed her conceptual framework to reflect the image of nursing, it was in order to provide a clear structure for nurses to carry out their care for patients and a rationale for this care. She devised a model of *living* on which to base her model for *nursing*, on the assumption that most individuals require nursing care only occasionally in their lifetime, so that nursing should reflect the patient's model for living and so cause minimal disruption in his life.

The model of living, originally composed of sixteen 'activities of daily living' (ADLs), was based on the concept of human needs: a brief outline of the characteristics of this theory was given in the previous chapter. Abraham Maslow, a pioneer of humanistic

13

psychology, proposed in 1954 a hierarchy of needs as a source of human motivation, asserting that the needs that are low in the hierarchy must be satisfied before the higher needs can become significant forces for motivation. He orders his list of needs as follows:

- physiological needs;
- safety needs;
- needs for love and belonging;
- self-esteem needs;
- learning, or cognitive needs;
- aesthetic needs;
- self-actualization needs.

(Maslow 1954)

These are typically represented as a diagram to clarify the hierarchical structure of human needs (Figure 2.1).

Figure 2.1 *The hierarchy of human needs (Maslow 1954)*

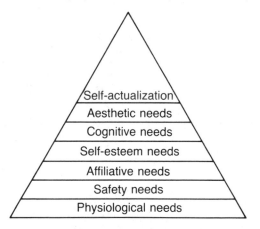

From this concept, Virginia Henderson (1969) identified fourteen universal human needs, which were adopted by the International Council of Nurses. The needs may be paraphrased thus:

- to breathe normally;
- to eat and drink adequately;
- to eliminate body waste;
- to move and maintain desirable posture;
- to sleep and rest;
- to select suitable clothes, to dress and undress;
- to maintain body temperature;

- to keep the body clean and protect skin;
- to avoid dangers and to avoid injury to others;
- to communicate with others, to express emotions;
- to worship according to one's faith;
- to work in such a way that a sense of achievement is experienced;
- to participate in recreation;
- to learn, discover and satisfy curiosity as part of normal develop ment.

This concept of nursing based on helping an individual to satisfy his basic human needs influenced the development of the Roper–Logan–Tierney model, but it was the passivity inherent in the concept of needs which led Roper to translate them into the original list of sixteen ADLs (Roper 1976).

To emphasise further the *active* element of her model, all the activities were specified as verbs, such as 'mobilising' rather than 'mobility'. She divided these activities into those that are essential for life, equating with Maslow's physical and safety needs, and those that enhance the quality of life, corresponding with Maslow's needs for love, self-esteem, learning, beauty and self-fulfilment. Roper also added 'dying' to her list of ADLs, as the last activity in everyone's life. Later, in 1976, together with Logan and Tierney, work started on *The Elements of Nursing* (published in 1980), in which the model was refined to its present form.

KEY CONCEPTS IN THE MODEL

The nature of the individual

In this model man is seen as engaging in a process of living from conception to death, and continually changing and developing through this life span. During his life span man carries out different types of activities, described as 'activities of living' (ALs). Although all of these activities overlap and cannot be isolated, it is helpful to describe them separately (pages 20–3). (The twelve ALs were redefined from the original sixteen ADLs as it was recognised that not every activity was carried out on a daily basis.) Each activity is seen being influenced by physical, emotional, sociocultural and economic factors, and man's uniqueness is expressed in the individual way in which he carries out each living activity. All the other activities that an individual carries out during his life span are described in the early work of Roper, Logan and Tierney as the comforting, preventing and seeking activities. 'Comforting' activi-

15

ties include such activities as going to bed early with a good book and a tot of whisky when you feel miserable at the start of a cold, while an example of a 'preventing' activity is to avoid people with colds to try to prevent yourself getting into this position in the first place. 'Seeking' activities include such activities as seeking knowledge by reading or educational pursuits, or seeking help when you acknowledge the need for it. These activities are influenced by the same factors that influence the ALs, and demonstrate the same individuality in the way in which they are carried out. They are not described in the later version of the model.

Related to the individual's life span is a dependence–independence continuum. This acknowledges the fact that there are times in life when an individual cannot carry out every activity independently; it may be related to age – for example a baby is totally dependent in nearly every activity – or dependence may be caused by illness, injury, congenital or acquired disability, pathological or degenerative changes, or infection. Emotional, social or economic reasons may also contribute to a change in dependence or independence, for example a depressed person may not be motivated to eat or wash, while lack of money or resources may decrease independence in leisure or working activities.

From this description of the beliefs and values about the nature of man, five major components of the model have been identified:

- activities of living, and activities of comforting, preventing and seeking;
- the life span;
- the independence–dependence continuum;
- factors influencing the ALs;
- individuality in carrying out the ALs.

The next chapter shows how the model for nursing is based on these five components of the model for living.

Health and illness

Health is difficult to define because like most concepts it may have a different meaning for each individual, even among those sharing the same culture. Roper, Logan and Tierney believe that it can only be defined in relation to the individual, taking into consideration personal expectation and the level of functioning in ordinary living; they see no clear boundary between health and illness.

The goal of all health care, and therefore of nursing in any model, may be defined in broad terms as helping the patient to retain or regain health, or to adapt to a changed health status. Thus the goal of nursing is dependent on the model's definition of the concept of health. The goals of *nursing* in the model are concerned with the patient's goals for *living*; they seek to cause minimal disruption to the usual process of living, and are based on an individual maintaining or regaining independence in the activities of living, or coping with a change in dependence–independence. The Roper–Logan–Tierney model is concerned not only with activities to meet the basic human needs, but also the individual way in which the activities are performed and the way in which people are educated or socialised to meet their needs.

Although in this model there is no clearly expressed definition of health, it appears that in the terms of the model's principles health is viewed as the ability to carry out the activities of living in a manner acceptable to the individual and the society in which he lives, and without causing harm to himself or others (subject to present knowledge and beliefs), in order to meet his basic human needs. It is also viewed as successfully coping with the difficulties in living, or with the subsequent needs to adapt to differing degrees of dependence.

The role of nursing in health and illness

Roper defined nursing as follows:

> Within the context of a health-care system and in a variety of combinations nursing is helping a person towards his personal independent pole of the continuum of each Activity of Daily Living; helping him to remain there; helping him to cope with any movement towards the dependent poles; in some instances encouraging him to move towards the dependent pole or poles; and because man is finite, helping him to die with dignity. (Roper 1976)

A later definition includes the idea of nursing as a discipline working within an organization:

> Nursing is directly or indirectly enabling each person in a health-care system to acquire, maintain or restore his maximum level of self-care/independence; or to cope with being dependent in any of his activities of daily living. Nursing incorporates co-ordination of help from other

17

health-care professions and at patient level it entails the performance of nursing activities from one or more of four groups of components of nursing. (Roper 1979)

In later writings Roper, Logan and Tierney describe the role of the nurse incorporating the concept of health and illness. Nursing is described as helping patients to prevent, solve, alleviate or cope with actual or potential problems related to the activities of living. They describe nurses in an independent practitioner role when carrying out the comforting component of nursing, in a dependent role when carrying out care prescribed by doctors or other health professionals, and in a role which may be independent or interdependent when carrying out the preventive component, emphasising the role of the nurse as part of the team concerned with health and health education (Roper *et al.* 1985). Figure 2.2 depicts these roles.

Figure 2.2 *Examples of nursing roles in a 24-hour period, related to ALs, the life span and the independence–dependence continuum*

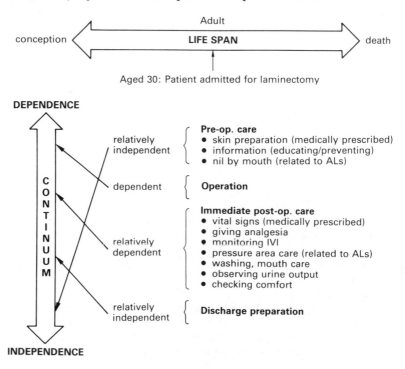

18

The environment

The authors refer to the environment in relation to the influence on each activity of living but do not define it specifically. They make no distinction between internal and external environment but they describe physiological and psychological factors that influence each AL, as well as social, economic and political factors which indicate that ALs are influenced by an internal and an external environment. The key concepts will be discussed more fully in the critique in Part III.

The five components (page 16) of the model for living are the basis for nursing care in the model for nursing. In conjunction with the care directly related to the ALs, nurses also carry out comforting, preventing and medically-prescribed activities. Comforting activities, readily recognised by all nurses but too numerous to describe, include all the nurse-initiated care planned to increase the patient's physical or emotional comfort. Preventing activities include those to prevent potential problems becoming actual problems, such as complications of bed rest, and may be initiated by the nurse alone or with another health professional. Preventive activities may include health education. Medically-prescriptive activities include those prescribed by medical or other professionals but carried out by nurses, in response to the seeking-help activities of the patient. Although all of these activities may be directly related to specific ALs this may not be obvious, so the flexibility of the model makes it unnecessary to try to categorise all nursing care or all patient problems under the heading of an activity of living; indeed to do so may look unnatural or contrived. In the following chapter all five components are described in depth, and in the context of the nursing process.

CHAPTER THREE

The components of the model and the nursing process

ACTIVITIES OF LIVING

The twelve activities of living identified in the model are maintaining a safe environment, communicating, breathing, eating and drinking, eliminating, personal cleansing and dressing, controlling body temperature, mobilising, working and playing, expressing sexuality, sleeping, and dying.

Maintaining a safe environment

This AL includes all those activities necessary to protect oneself and one's family, such as preventing accidents and infection at home or in the workplace, or, on a more global level, buying products that will not pollute the environment, for example. When a person requires nursing care his ability to maintain his own safety must be assessed in the context of his illness, treatment, dependence–independence status, position on the life span, and a new environment or routine.

Communication

Communication is an essential part of social interaction: it includes communication by all means – writing, reading, talking, and all forms of non-verbal communication. Problems with communicating may have physical causes, such as impairments of speech, hearing or sight; there may be psychological or intellectual reasons; or there may be cultural or language difficulties.

Subjective feelings, attitudes, anxieties and pain are all communicated, verbally or non-verbally, consciously or subconsciously, so pain as a problem, unless obviously related to some other AL, is included under this heading.

Breathing

Breathing is obviously the most vital activity, but when it is effortless and problem-free, it is one which every individual can carry out independently irrespective of age.

Eating and drinking

This AL includes not only the physical acts of eating or drinking but also the activity of obtaining and preparing food. Problems may therefore include physical ones related to chewing, swallowing, self-feeding, the ability to reach the shops or to cook; psychological or intellectual difficulties concerned with knowledge or motivation (eating and drinking may be a comforting activity, as well as an essential living activity, in times of unhappiness or stress); or socioeconomic problems of availability of resources. It will be readily seen that problems in mobilising, for example, may affect the ability to carrying out this activity effectively – one example of the activities being interrelated.

Eliminating

An essential activity of living in which problems may cause enormous inconvenience, pain, embarrassment and misery. Problems may be caused by limited mobility, making it difficult to manage to get to the lavatory and to manage independently. Urinary tract infections may cause problems of acute discomfort and pain, while even a minor degree of incontinence will cause inconvenience and embarrassment, even leading to social withdrawal. Clearly this activity is also interrelated with mobility, expressing sexuality, eating and drinking, personal cleansing and dressing, and working and playing.

Personal cleansing and dressing

This AL includes the physical acts of carrying out these activities; it also includes the condition of the skin, so pressure-area care is included in this AL. Some nurses feel that pressure-area care could be included in maintaining a safe environment or mobilising – an opinion which again illustrates the interdependence of the activities – but the model literature places it clearly in this AL. Clothing and hairstyles may reflect cultural, social, economic and sexual aspects of an individual, so this activity is closely related not only to mobilising and controlling body temperature, but also to communicating, expressing sexuality, and working and playing. Problems may occur in any aspect of the activity, but not all are amenable to nursing intervention.

Controlling body temperature

This is one of those essential activities about which we never think until a problem occurs. In very young babies and the elderly, the heat-regulating system is less efficient, but on the whole people cope with changes in environmental temperature by adding or removing clothing. Pyrexia and hypothermia represent the two extremes of problems in this activity.

Mobilising

'Mobilising' is described by Roper, Logan and Tierney as a 'clumsy but explicit' word for this activity. Problems are frequently encountered and readily recognised by nurses in all areas of practice, and when mobilising includes every muscular movement, large or small, it is easy to see how mobilising problems may affect every other activity.

Working and playing

These take up a large proportion of the waking hours of an individual, although often it feels as though there is a preponderance of the working component! Both may involve physical or intellectual activity, both may include comforting and seeking activities, and both may contribute to health or illness. Examples include exercise, which stimulates circulation and a sense of well-being but may also cause injuries, while a degree of stress in a demanding job may be necessary for motivation but may become harmful when experienced to excess.

As all nurses know, the fact of being ill or in hospital, or away from the normal working routine, sometimes causes problems in itself, such as anxiety about separation from family and friends or about the large backlog of work which will accumulate in one's absence. Sometimes there is little that a nurse can do about these problems but it is still essential to be aware of their possible existence.

Expressing sexuality

This includes aspects of femininity and masculinity, body image, and the way in which an individual perceives himself or herself in general. Any problems directly related to sexual organs or function would be included in this AL, in addition to problems of altered body image, both actual and perceived.

Stuart (1953) quotes:

> All damage to the body is first and foremost damage to the self and there is no really good treatment which does not take into account the primary necessity for healing and establishing the ego, for making the self picture whole again. (Chapman 1982)

Sleeping

An activity (in the broadest sense of the word) which takes up to about one-third of our lives, though this often does not seem enough. The amount of sleep required varies between individuals, with babies often sleeping most of the 24 hours (so the books say) and, at the other end of the life span, the elderly taking frequent short naps. Young adults are usually able to sleep till very late in the morning while young children wake very early but are never ready for bed in the evening. Some people sleep in armchairs all the evening, waking only to get ready for bed for some more sleep; others toss and turn till the early hours. From a nursing point of view it is useful to know the usual sleeping pattern of a patient in order to know how his illness is affecting his sleep. Sleep may be disturbed by almost any problem which affects any other activity of living.

Dying

The last activity of living that anyone will perform, and all the other living activities may be concerned with the process of dying. Problems with this activity will include those associated with the individual who is dying and also those with relatives and friends who are grieving.

As this list shows, it is impossible in practice to separate the ALs from the other activities, except in theoretical discussion. To apply the nursing model in practice requires knowledge of the physiological and psychosocial aspects of each AL, in addition to professional, technological and interpersonal skills to perform the care.

This list suggests a systems-theory approach, with the physical activities representing biological systems whose interdependence is reflected in the relationship of each activity to others.

THE LIFE SPAN

The life span extends from conception to death, but although conception is represented on the life span birth is not identified as an activity of living, as Roper, Logan and Tierney acknowledge but do not explain. Apart from this no identifiable stages are plotted on the life span, although eight developmental life stages are described in the model literature. These stages are:

- prenatal (conception to birth);
- infancy (birth to 5 years);
- childhood (6 to 12 years);
- adolescence (13 to 18 years);
- early adulthood (19 to 30 years);
- middle years (31 to 45 years);
- late adulthood (46 to 65 years);
- old age (66 plus).

The stages identified are very similar to those of Erikson (1950), the only major developmental theorist to propose a life-span approach. Erikson identified eight psychosocial stages from birth to old age, each stage presenting a 'task' or 'dilemma' for the individual to resolve. In the first stage, for example, the task of the baby is to develop trust in his mother (or carer). The degree of success in resolving each dilemma as it arises will influence the ability to cope with the next stage, and ultimately affect the overall psychosocial well-being and the further development of the individual (Bee and Mitchell 1980).

Erikson also acknowledges the importance of biological and experiential influences on development, which are reflected in the account of physical, intellectual, emotional and social development across the life stages described in the Roper–Logan–Tierney model. In doing this, the model also draws on the cognitive developmental theories of Piaget, the psychosexual theories of Freud, and the work

24

of Bowlby on child care (Roper *et al.* 1985). To apply the model in practice, nurses' knowledge must include awareness of developmental stages and the health problems related to them.

THE DEPENDENCE–INDEPENDENCE CONTINUUM

The model recognises that there cannot be a fixed point on the continuum at which to assess the dependence/independence status for an individual: dependence must be assessed in every activity of living when the need for nursing is acknowledged. For example, a patient who is totally dependent on others for mobilising may be independent in communicating and breathing but require a certain amount of help with eliminating, with eating and drinking and with personal cleansing and dressing. The two opposing poles of total dependence and independence are identified but there are no measurable points between. For each AL, criteria by which the degree of dependence may be assessed must be defined by the nurse based on clinical, developmental and social norms, taking into account also the individuality of the patient. These judgements cannot be made with exactitude and it may be hard to compare the dependence of the patient at one point with his dependence at a later stage of recovery.

FACTORS INFLUENCING ACTIVITIES OF LIVING

Five groups of factors are identified in the model for living as influencing the way in which any individual performs the living activities:

- physical factors;
- psychological factors;
- sociocultural factors;
- environmental factors;
- politico-economic factors.

Each AL may be influenced to a greater or lesser extent by any one of these factors. The activity of eating and drinking is the example used in the model literature to explain this feature (Roper *et al.* 1985).

As the term 'activity' implies, physical influences are readily identifiable in all ALs and, with the exception of a deeply uncon-

25

scious patient, the psychological influences are also well recognised. Sociocultural factors influence our communication, eating and drinking, hygiene activities, the way we dress, work and play, our sexual activities, and the rites associated with dying. Environmental factors, such as climate, for example, influence nearly every AL; with increased ecological awareness, the influence becomes even more extensive. Political and economic factors such as wealth and poverty affect the resources required to carry out living activities; they are easily recognised by their influence on what we eat, the clothes we wear and the leisure activities we pursue, to mention just three examples.

INDIVIDUALITY

In this model of nursing it is the individual way in which each person carries out each activity that provides the basis for planned individual care. Individuality as a component of the model is dependent on all the other components, emphasising the interdependence of all parts of the model. Individuality is influenced by the age of the individual (where he is on the life span) and the extent to which he can carry out the activity independently (where he is on the dependence–independence continuum). It is also influenced, of course, by the factors described above. The questions that must be asked to assess a person's individuality will address the issues of how, how often, why, when and where each activity is performed, and will also consider the person's knowledge, beliefs and attitudes about each activity. These are central to our individuality.

The relationships between the model components are illustrated in Figure 3.1.

THE MODEL AND THE NURSING PROCESS

Assessing

The term 'assessing' is used in the Roper–Logan–Tierney model to describe the first stage of the nursing process, emphasising that this is an active process, and not a once-only event. It consists of collecting and reviewing information about the patient and identifying any problems, actual or potential, which are amenable to nursing intervention.

26

Figure 3.1 *A model for living*

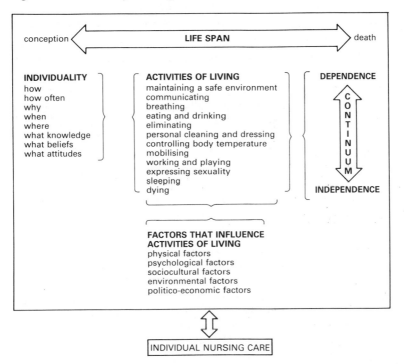

Collecting and reviewing information

The model provides a structure for collecting appropriate information which helps to build up a picture of the whole individual. Some of the information will be biographical, including clinical observations, but the greater part will be related to the ALs. This framework allows the nurse to collect information about the way in which each activity is carried out normally, in order to provide a baseline against which to measure the change in the independence–dependence status of the patient.

The questions 'How?', 'How often?', 'When?' and so on provide an *aide-mémoire* for assessing, and when addressed help to build up a comprehensive picture of the way in which any AL is carried out. There are occasions when it seems superfluous, or even intrusive, to ask a patient questions about an AL. For example, it may seem unnecessary to enquire about the bowel pattern of an otherwise healthy young man being admitted for elective orthopaedic surgery.

However, addressing a few questions to him may allow a picture to emerge which reveals not only how often he has his bowels open but also the extent of his knowledge or anxieties about this function. This could become very useful if problems were to occur after surgery and would provide a base on which to plan his care. Similarly, when confronted by an articulate, appropriately dressed patient walking briskly into the ward with no apparent breathing problems, it might be tempting to omit a few ALs from the assessment, to save precious time. Roper *et al.* state that in some circumstances it is not necessary to consider every AL for every patient assessment (Roper *et al.* 1983). However my own view is that, with the exception of 'dying', every AL *should* be considered, albeit briefly and without urgency, if appropriate then recording a statement to the effect that there are no apparent problems with the AL. Quality of nursing care can only be measured if it can be observed, and an omission in the records may indicate an omission of care in any stage of the nursing process.

On the question of the AL 'dying', as it is an activity carried out only once, there are numerous situations in which assessment would be highly inappropriate. This must be left to the professional judgement of the nurse in every case, a fact that emphasises the skills required in assessment.

Identifying the problems

In addition to problems associated with the ALs, which are usually readily recognised by the patient, there are other complications that may or may not be experienced by the patient as problems, such as wounds, cardiac monitors, intravenous infusions, or blood-glucose tests. These are described in the model as 'problems derived from medical (or other health professional) prescription'. Categorising and recording these and potential problems within the model seems often to cause nurses consternation, yet they do fit well in the context of the model's principles.

Medically-derived problems such as those described above require nursing intervention, to maintain or to give the treatment prescribed by other professionals and to help the patient to carry out his usual activities while the problem exists. This nursing care makes up the 'medically-prescriptive' component of nursing defined in the model. Although the ALs are the main focus of nursing actions, reflecting the unique role of the nurse in comforting, helping, teaching and preventive modes, the medically-prescriptive component constitutes what McFarlane (1980) calls the 'collaborative' role of the nurse, developed in the model for nursing from the seeking activities outlined in the model for living.

The nursing world sometimes seems to be divided into nurses who record all the potential problems under the sun and those who record none. A 'problem' may be simply defined as *the difference between a situation as it is and as one would like it to be*. Assessing each AL reveals that this is the difference between how the patient would usually be able to, or wish to, perform the activity of living and how he is able to do so at the time of assessment. Although the patient may not identify potential problems in this way, clinical, physiological and psychosocial knowledge will lead the nurse to do so, and to determine the appropriate nursing action required to prevent these *potential* problems becoming *actual* problems. Some potential problems are not amenable to nursing care, of course, in which case the nurse may decide to seek the help of other professionals or the family; in other cases quiet observation is all that is required. Each potential problem should be *recorded*, but it will not always require a care plan. Because it makes the question of potential problems explicit the model may be applied to nursing in health, as well as in illness: this emphasises the preventive aspect of nursing care.

Based as it is on a theory of needs, the physical activities categorised as essential must be seen to be carried out effectively before others are assessed. The order of priority in which the ALs should be assessed is exactly that which presents itself with each individual patient.

As each activity of living is assessed, the developmental stage of the patient must be considered (which requires knowledge of normal development); and for each activity some measure of independence or dependence must be established, and the factors influencing it taken into account.

Planning the care

This stage of the nursing process includes setting goals and selecting nursing actions to attain these goals. This activity aims to help the patient to prevent, solve, and alleviate problems, or to cope with those that cannot be prevented, solved or alleviated. Goals of nursing care must be realistic and achievable and reflect the patient's goals for living, so they must be set in close partnership with the patient and based on assessment of the individual ALs and on the nursing knowledge associated with them. Goals must be related to the place of the patient on the independence–dependence continuum in any one AL, and must identify the movement to be achieved along the continuum. They must also be observable and measurable, to provide a link with the evaluation stage of the process – results that cannot be observed or measured cannot be evaluated. The difference between short- and long-term goals is acknowledged in the model, and short-term goals, with clear indications of the timeframe in which they should be achieved, are preferred.

Bond (1984) believes, and I am sure most nurses would agree, that it is nurses in short-term care settings who find goal-setting most difficult, in particular in emergency situations or those which change very rapidly, such as during recovery after an operation. In these cases, whatever the model in use, the goals cannot always be agreed with the patient, and often they cannot be recorded or evaluated as they are achieved or not achieved. But the nursing process is still happening and the model principles may still be observed in practice. Using a nursing model within the nursing process is more than a paper exercise!

Problems in one activity of living may involve several others, as explained on pages 20–3. For example, if a patient has a problem sleeping, a goal to achieve six hours' sleep per night might require additional goals and nursing actions related to all the other activities.

The planning and recording of care are means of communicating with other nurses involved. Plans and records should include as much detail as is practical, so that other nurses can continue the care.

Implementing the care

Nursing care is focused on the usual ways in which the patient carries out ALs: the intention is to cause minimal disruption. For example, a person unable to cope independently with the AL of personal cleansing and dressing, who usually has a daily bath, may be helped to continue this in hospital, if his condition allows, or alternatively may be given a daily bed bath. This care may be described as the comforting, or nurse-initiated, component of care. Sometimes, however, the usual ways of carrying out activities may have contributed to the health problem, as in an unsuitable diet which has caused obesity: in this case the focus would still be the AL of eating and drinking, but the component of nursing care would be preventive and aimed at re-educating the patient into different ways of eating.

Nursing care derived from medical prescription does not primarily focus on, but may generate problems in, a specific AL. An intravenous infusion, prescribed by a doctor and requiring care given by nurses, may cause practical difficulties in washing, mobilising, eliminating or sleeping, any or all of which may require nursing intervention.

Evaluating the care

Evaluating, the fourth stage of the nursing process, is directly linked with the planning stage and may be defined simply as determining the extent to which the goals have been achieved. Goals related to ALs may be evaluated by the extent of movement towards the independent pole of the continuum, or by the adjustment made by the patient to increasing dependence. Other goals may be evaluated by measurement, such as weight loss in the overweight patient, or the reduced diameter of a leg ulcer, or an increase in blood-glucose estimation in a hypoglycaemic patient. Even goals which seem difficult to measure, such as adapting to an altered body image, may be evaluated by the extent to which the patient has achieved the goals of looking at the affected part of his body, talking about it, touching it and caring for it. This stage of the nursing process is the stepping stone for reassessment, for re-examining and modifying the problem statements, the goals and goal dates, and the care that has been given. Figure 3.2 offers a diagrammatic representation.

SUMMARY

In this chapter, the five components of the model have been described in detail and in relation to one another, demonstrating the model's logical and systematic structure, and the concept of holism (see Figure 3.1). It has been shown that the model may be applied in health and illness and may be used in preventive health education. It takes into consideration all the factors that influence our lives, and deals with the sometimes neglected activity of dying. The model may be used logically within the framework of the nursing process, allowing flexibility and scope for professional judgement.

Figure 3.2 *The model and the nursing process*

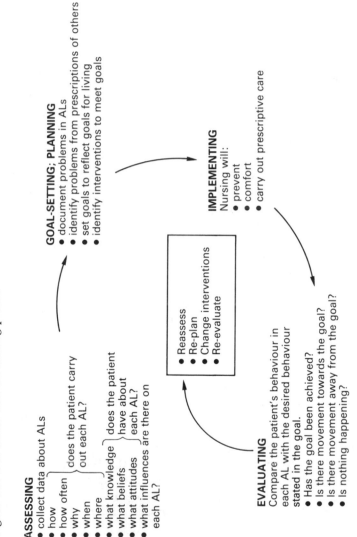

ASSESSING
- collect data about ALs
- how
- how often ⎫ does the patient carry
- why ⎬ out each AL?
- when
- where
- what knowledge ⎫ does the patient
- what beliefs ⎬ have about
- what attitudes ⎭ each AL?
- what influences are there on each AL?

GOAL-SETTING; PLANNING
- document problems in ALs
- identify problems from prescriptions of others
- set goals to reflect goals for living
- identify interventions to meet goals

IMPLEMENTING
Nursing will:
- prevent
- comfort
- carry out prescriptive care

EVALUATING
Compare the patient's behaviour in each AL with the desired behaviour stated in the goal.
- Has the goal been achieved?
- Is there movement towards the goal?
- Is there movement away from the goal?
- Is nothing happening?

- Reassess
- Re-plan
- Change interventions
- Re-evaluate

PART II

Applying the model

CHAPTER FOUR

Care study: a patient undergoing major bowel surgery

This care study describes the nursing care given to a middle-aged lady on a surgical ward from the time of admission to the ward until her discharge fifteen days later. Events leading up to her admission are described briefly to provide a background to the study.

The patient's nursing care is described in detail under the headings of the activities of living and within the stages of the nursing process, but details of the medical care are included only if directly relevant to the nursing care. The different components of nursing care are identified. For ease of presentation the planning, implementation and evaluation of the care are subdivided into pre-operative and post-operative stages, and are described in the text and by means of a care plan.

MRS MARGARET WELLS

Three months prior to admission Mrs Wells had noticed that her bowel pattern had changed, with alternating bouts of diarrhoea and constipation. At first she had felt mildly worried but had thought it would pass; five weeks prior to admission, however, she had noticed some blood in her stools during a bout of diarrhoea. She consulted her own GP, who referred her to the surgical consultant. A colonoscopy revealed an annular carcinoma at the flexure of the sigmoid colon. Two weeks later she was admitted as a planned admission for resection of the sigmoid colon, and formation of a colostomy as a temporary measure to allow the anastomosis to heal.

35

ADMISSION

The setting for the care study

The setting for this care study is a thirty-bedded mixed-sex surgical ward, consisting of four four-bedded bays, one eight-bedded bay and six *en suite* single rooms. Team nursing is used, and patients are allocated in each shift to teams of nurses each taking a different area of the ward. The ward supports first- and third-year learners; on average there are eight nurses (including learners) on an early shift, four on a late shift and four on night duty.

Assessing on admission

Margaret was admitted during the afternoon of 5 May, two weeks after her colonoscopy. She was accompanied by her husband. She was a fit-looking 53-year-old lady, of medium height, and smart, casual appearance.

She was shown to her single room by a staff nurse who introduced herself and established that Margaret would like to be called by her first name. The purpose of assessment was explained but as her husband could only stay a short time it was decided that it could be delayed until after she had organised herself and her husband had left. (It would obviously not always be realistic to leave assessment until later but it is not always necessary to do it at once.) Information was given about visiting hours, ward facilities and the storing of valuables. Margaret asked about smoking and was told that she could smoke in the day-room.

By way of an introduction to assessing, information obtained from the medical notes was confirmed (Figure 4.1, page 56). This approach helps to put the patient at ease because these questions are expected. Most patients also expect to be asked questions related to occupation, religion, appetite, elimination, and sleep, whatever the focus of their problems, in addition to being weighed, asked for a urine specimen, and having their temperature taken. Questions related to other activities of living may appear irrelevant or intrusive to the patient, and must therefore be handled with sensitivity.

Assessing is described below in the order in which ALs are usually listed, but information is usually collected in an informal semi-structured interview with the headings used only as prompts. The completed assessment is shown in Figure 4.2 (page 57).

36

Maintaining a safe environment

Margaret had already established that she was a smoker; the hospital's safety rules had been explained. Although normally independent, there would be a period while in the theatre and immediately after when Margaret would be dependent on the care of others. She had no dentures or loose teeth. The potential problem of complications of surgery was identified.

Communicating

Margaret was articulate, with no speech, sensory or hearing problems; she wore glasses for reading only. She was asked whether she felt clear about the reasons for her admission and operation and indicated that although the surgeon had told her that she had 'an ulcer in the bowl' she herself suspected cancer and her own GP had confirmed this. She said she understood the colostomy in theory but was unable to imagine what it would look like. She had talked about it to her husband. Being able to predict the duration of stressful situations seems to reduce anxiety, and it seemed that the temporary nature of the colostomy was helping her to cope at this stage (Hilgarde *et al.* 1979). Wilson Barnett (1978a) suggests that anxiety is at its greatest within the first twenty-four hours of admission but may not necessarily be expressed as such, so despite Margaret's fairly calm exterior, anxiety about the operation and its effects was identified as a potential problem.

Breathing

Although Margaret had been a smoker for over thirty years she normally had no breathing problems or chest pain. She smoked about ten cigarettes a day and had never smoked more. The potential problem of breathing difficulties after anaesthetic was identified.

Eating and drinking

Normally Margaret had a good appetite, with no particular dislikes. She described a well-balanced diet, and said that she was usually about half a stone heavier than she would like to be, so that she occasionally tried to diet. She estimated that she had lost about half a stone in weight in the last three months during the time her appetite had decreased. She was a social drinker who kept within what she believed to be the 'safe limits' for a woman. The potential problem of change in diet to suit her different elimination needs after surgery was identified, in addition to the actual problem of loss of appetite and the change in eating and drinking before and immediately following the operation. Margaret's weight on admission was 62 kg (9 st. 10 lb.).

Eliminating

In view of the reason for admission this activity was the focus of the problem for Margaret; she answered questions freely, concentrating on functional rather than aesthetic aspects. It seemed important that she should have the opportunity to discuss how she felt about the formation of a stoma or to ask questions related to it, but this proved to be fairly difficult. She maintained a 'stiff upper lip' attitude, indicating that she would 'cope with it when it happens, so there's no need to dwell on it now'. Although nothing was recorded, difficulty with adaptation to the stoma was borne in mind as a potential problem. Margaret had had no previous problems with bowel function and experienced a regular daily pattern. Similarly there had been no problems with urinary eliminating: she sometimes had to pass urine once during the night, and did so about four-hourly during the day.

She commented that she would be relieved when 'it's all dealt with'. As she would return from theatre with a urinary catheter and a colostomy the change in mode of elimination was identified as an actual problem. Ward urinalysis revealed no abnormalities.

Personal cleansing and dressing

Margaret's clean, attractive appearance showed that there were no obvious problems with independence in this activity. She revealed that her younger daughter was a hairdresser and 'kept her up to date'. Although a thorough examination of Margaret's skin was not carried out, there were no visible lesions or bruising and she said that she had no skin problems or scars from previous operations. In the model pressure-area and wound care are considered under this heading, so wound infection was identified as a potential problem. In view of Margaret's good skin condition and a Norton score of 20 on admission, pressure-area risk was recorded as a potential problem but no care plan was made at this stage even though Margaret would be less active than usual for a few days. For a short period post-operatively Margaret would need help with personal hygiene, so that was identified as an actual problem.

Controlling body temperature

Margaret's temperature on admission was 36.4 °C. No problem was identified; regular observations would be carried out after the operation in order to identify any increase in temperature as a possible indication of infection.

Mobilising

Margaret was fully independent on admission, but due to constraints imposed by treatment and her own physical condition her ability to mobilise would be limited after her operation. Complications of bed rest have been recognised since the 1950s and have constituted a preventive component of nursing since 1963 (Roper 1976). This had already been identified as a potential problem. Possible complications include chest infection, deep vein thrombosis, pulmonary embolism, and pressure-area skin damage.

Working and playing

Margaret had worked as a part-time dental receptionist for ten years, enjoying her job. She lived with her husband and younger daughter, and also had a married daughter and a 3-year-old grandson. Leisure activities included amateur dramatics, church pursuits and social outings. Apart from swimming during holidays and walking she took no regular exercise.

Margaret might feel isolated in a single room and loneliness at separation from her husband and family might be a potential problem. Research by Wilson Barnett (1978b) demonstrated that absence from family or even from work can cause distress for hospital patients, in addition to the anxiety about procedures and outcomes which are well recognised.

Expressing sexuality

It was obvious that Margaret took trouble with her personal appearance, but in this initial assessment she expressed no feelings about the effect of surgery on her appearance or on her relationship with her husband so the subject was not explored. She had not menstruated for two years. Woods and Mandetta (1975) claim that body image develops from a person's experience of her own body: when this is altered, with the possible loss of control of a function, there may be feelings of unacceptability which affect self-esteem and perceived sexual attractiveness. In addition, Golden (1980) asserts that a high percentage of patients experience sexual difficulties after stoma surgery, while Ainslie (1981) has shown that even the *diagnosis* of cancer alters the perception of body image. In view of these findings an altered body image was identified as an actual problem.

Sleeping

Margaret said that she usually woke once or twice in the night but never felt ready to wake in the morning. On average she went to bed at about 22.00 and rose at 06.45. She had never taken any sleeping tablets but had recently considered asking for some. An actual problem of anxiety about her sleeping pattern was identified.

Dying

In view of Margaret's diagnosis and the anxiety this usually causes, oblique or overt reference to prognosis or mortality might have been expected: no such reference was made, however, and her silence was respected. It was important to keep in mind that Margaret and her family might feel the need of help or support related to aspects of dying.

PRE-OPERATIVE CARE

A list of actual and potential problems may be seen in the assessment form (Figure 4.2, page 57).

Description of the nursing care Much of the pre-operative care is preventive and derived from medical prescription. It is not always appropriate to have goals closely allied to goals for living as they are usually very different from usual activities. A large proportion of the nursing care is also concerned with emotional care: at the care-planning stage Margaret was still at the independent end of the dependence–independence continuum.

Communicating

Problem   Potential anxiety about illness and treatment (not openly expressed).

Setting goals   Long- and short-term goals have already been discussed (page 30). A long-term goal is usually expressed in terms similar to those in which the problem is expressed, while the short-term goals are expressed as observable and measurable signs that can be used to evaluate the extent to which the long-term goal is being achieved. If possible a time by which the goals should be met should be stated.

In this case, where Margaret might be anxious but had not said so, the long-term goal was for her to feel less anxious: a short-term goal set to achieve this was for her to be able to discuss any fears, by the day of her operation, so that they might be relieved. This would also show that she was able to trust the nurses enough to be open about her fears. Rogers (1951) asserts that the essential qualities to encourage trust are empathy, being genuine, and showing 'unconditional positive regard'. Janis (1983) also suggests that a nurse should concentrate on building a relationship, in which as soon as possible she becomes for the patient a significant person with influence, in order to encourage compliance and motivation for recovery. With problems affecting feelings there can be no rigid rules, but results from several research studies have shown that information given to, and understood by, patients prior to operations and investigations can help to reduce anxiety and aid recovery (Hayward 1978; Boore 1978). So another short-term goal was that by the day of surgery Margaret (and possibly her husband) would have demonstrated understanding of the reasons for, and the nature of, the operation and the care she was to be given.

Nursing actions and evaluation   Nursing actions were focused on information-giving and relationship-building. Margaret was given information regarding the time and date of her operation; the visits of the anaesthetist, the physiotherapist and the stoma nurse; the bowel preparation and diet regime; and what to expect after the operation. The staff nurse remained with her while she was examined by a doctor, and checked her understanding of what she had been told. By the way she was able to discuss it in her own words Margaret showed understanding of all the information, but despite privacy and the opportunity to ask questions or talk, she did not do so.

Eating and drinking; eliminating

Problem 1 Alteration in eating and drinking before and after the operation. The potential problem of inhaling food during the operation.

Problem 2 Alteration in the mode of eliminating following the operation.

Setting goals The long-term goal was to have an empty stomach while in theatre (to prevent regurgitation or inhalation of food), and an empty bowel on which to operate. The short-term goal was to have a clear fluid result from the colonic lavage by the evening before the operation, which would indicate an empty bowel.

Nursing actions and evaluation The stoma nurse visited Margaret on the day after admission, identified a suitable site for the stoma, and showed her the appliances she would be using after the operation. Margaret handled these and said that although it was difficult to imagine she was sure she would manage.

Margaret was given nourishing fluids only for the following two days. These were strained soups and milk drinks as desired, as well as tea, coffee and fruit drinks. On the day before her operation she was given clear fluids only, including meat extracts, clear fruit juice and water. On the day of operation Margaret was allowed nothing by mouth for at least six hours before going to theatre. The reasons for this regime are that the stomach empties its contents into the duodenum 2–6 hours after a meal and it may take up to eighteen hours for the contents to reach the sigmoid colon (Tortora and Anagnostakos 1981). This was explained to Margaret. (Hamilton-Smith's study (1972) found that the fasting time was usually set for convenience and to establish a regime which helped to prevent mistakes rather than on the basis of scientific knowledge and individual need: she suggests that anxiety may slow down the process of digestion and this must be considered.) The 'nil by mouth from midnight' rule is in general use for morning operations, but Margaret was told that if she woke early she could ask for a drink. This was an individual decision of the night nurse. Knowing that one may have a drink is sometimes enough to relieve anxiety about this, but Margaret requested a drink at 03.45 and returned to sleep.

Margaret was also told that she would have an intravenous infusion on return from theatre, until she was able to start eating and drinking normally; a nasogastric tube, to prevent stomach secretions going to the bowel; and a urethral catheter on free drainage for a few days.

Margaret was given Bisocodyl 10 mg on the evenings of the 5th and 6th of May. This is a powerful bowel evacuant used before bowel surgery or investigations (ABPI 1981). The effects were explained and she was told that she would have colonic lavages during the evening prior to the operation to complete the process and to show that the bowel was empty. Her comment was, 'What an awful business this is turning out to be.' (There are other methods of achieving complete bowel evacuation but the method employed in this care study is widely used: see Peters 1983.) There was a clear result from the second lavage, during which Margaret became distressed and expressed feelings of disgust and revulsion and fears that she would never manage or be 'normal' again. At bedtime she was offered a sedative, Temazepam 20 mg, which she accepted, and she slept until 07.00.

Maintaining a safe environment

Problem Inability to maintain own safety in theatre or immediately post-op. Potential complications of surgery and bed rest.

The activities sometimes termed 'routine pre-op. care' are grouped together under this heading and include the elements of a pre-op. checklist (Figure 4.3, page 58). The pre-op. plan accompanied Margaret to theatre, with her medical notes and X-rays.

Setting goals Evaluation of the goals also acts as a check to ensure that all preparation has been carried out. The long-term goal is that the patient is safe in theatre and suffers no complications of surgery. Short-term goals included the following:

- that Margaret should understand the purpose of, and how to carry out, calf-muscle and breathing exercises;
- that her skin should be as free as possible from pathological micro-organisms;
- that any underlying clinical abnormalities should be identified so that they could be treated.

Nursing actions and evaluation On the morning before the operation Margaret's pubic and abdominal area was shaved, to make the skin as clean as possible to help prevent infection. This was explained to

43

Margaret. (There are conflicting opinions about the efficacy of this activity but the practice continues in some areas.) The nurse also checked that Margaret understood about the exercises. Calf-muscle exercises facilitate venous return by the massaging action on the leg vessels, while deep breathing causes maximum lung expansion which by a suction action facilitates venous return in the large vessels of the chest. Illingworth (1970) asserts that the period between 24 and 48 hours after surgery is most dangerous for the development of deep venous thrombosis, and the period between 7 and 14 days for pulmonary embolism. So it is important for the patient to understand *before*, and to do the exercises as soon as possible *after*, the operation.

On the morning of operation Margaret slept until after 07.00, after a drink in the early hours. She had a bath and dressed in a theatre gown, then returned to bed to read. Later the staff nurse, who had been on duty the previous evening, checked that Margaret had signed the 'consent to anaesthetic', that she was wearing her identity wristband, that she had no dentures in, and no make-up, nail varnish or jewellery on except her wedding ring, which was taped over. Her observations were recorded as follows: temperature 36 °C, pulse 82 beats, respirations 18 per minute. Her blood pressure was 135/85 mmHg.

Margaret suddenly asked a lot of questions about the operation and seemed worried about the after-effects of the anaesthetic. The staff nurse stayed for a time talking with her, and told her that she would return with the 'pre-med.' in about half an hour and would be with her when she went to theatre. Omnopon 20 mg with Scopolamine 0.4 mg was given intramuscularly at 10.15 after Margaret had been asked to empty her bladder and to remain in bed from then on. The effects of the pre-medication were explained and the nurse call-bell placed within reach. Margaret went to theatre at 11.05, awake but drowsy.

POST-OPERATIVE CARE

Margaret returned to the ward at 14.00 following the removal of an annular carcinoma, resection of the adjacent sections of the sigmoid colon, associated mesentery and immediate lymph drainage. Continuity of the bowel was restored by anastomosis of the remaining portions of the descending and sigmoid colon. A colostomy had been fashioned in the transverse colon, above the site of the anastomosis. Margaret had an intravenous infusion of dextrose in saline, running at a rate of 500 ml in six hours; a nasogastric tube and a urinary catheter, both on free drainage; a wound drain and a cellular dressing on the abdominal wound. Assessment established that Margaret was at the dependent pole of the continuum for most of the activities of living. As patients do not leave the recovery room until they are conscious, Margaret was able to breathe independently but even this activity required careful observation.

The assessment is shown in Figure 4.4 (page 61) and the care plan in Figure 4.5 (page 62).

Maintaining a safe environment

Setting goals   Some of the care had been planned with Margaret before the operation, but in the immediate post-operative period the priority of nursing care was to be able to identify the first signs of haemorrhage and shock associated with a lowered blood volume so that care related to all other activities of living would be on the basis of maintenance rather than active intervention. The primary goal of care in this period was that any bleeding that occurred would be promptly identified and dealt with. Specific goal standards stated that the pulse rate and blood pressure should return to their baseline readings within four hours of return to ward. (This standard is suitable only if the baseline rates are within the normal range for health.) Another observable goal was for Margaret's skin to remain pink and warm to the touch, an indication of adequate perfusion of oxygen to the tissues.

Nursing actions and evaluation   Pulse rate and blood pressure were recorded on return to the ward and then at half-hourly intervals until they had been recorded twice moving towards their pre-operative rate. They were then recorded hourly until they were stable at the baseline rate; from then on temperature, pulse and blood pressure were recorded four-hourly until they had remained within the normal range for the patient for 48 hours. Margaret made an uneventful recovery in the first six hours and at 19.00 her observations were as follows: temperature 37.6 °C; pulse 88 beats per minute; blood pressure 130/78 mmHg. There was no blood or exudate visible on her outer wound dressing; drainage from the wound drain was 150 ml, urinary drainage from the catheter was 100 ml; there was minimal bleeding from the stoma. The intravenous fluid was infusing at the prescribed rate.

Communicating

The second priority in this period was pain control. Roper *et al.* (1985) propose that pain that cannot logically be associated with any other activity of living should be considered as part of communicating. Although the pain after bowel surgery is clearly associated physiologically and structurally with eliminating, it is not subjectively perceived in this way at the time it is experienced, but is communicated either verbally or behaviourally. Roper quotes a definition of pain offered by McCaffery (1983): 'Pain is what the patient says it is, existing when he says it does.'

Setting goals   The long-term goal is relief of the pain, both for the comfort of the patient and to allow her to rest. Work done by Hans Selye (1976), the acknowledged authority on stress, established that conservation of energy is necessary for promotion of healing (Tortora and Anagnostakos 1981). Short-term goals were that the post-operative analgesia would relieve the pain within 20 minutes, that Margaret would be able to rest and remain reasonably comfortable during nursing activities and position changes, and that pain would decrease in intensity.

Nursing actions and evaluation   Pethidine 100 mg (analgesia) and Metoclopramide 10 mg (anti-emetic) were administered intramuscularly at 15.45. Margaret's face and hands were washed and her lips moistened but she was not disturbed further. She slept until 19.15 when she complained of pain and the dose was repeated. She was made more comfortable; she changed into her nightdress, rinsed her mouth with water and was given the call bell. She was told to ask for pain relief when she needed it, before the pain became severe. Before the operation the causes of pain and the principles of pain relief had been explained. A further two doses were given at 23.00 and at 05.00, with good effect. She was offered a mouthwash and her position was changed to relieve discomfort on each occasion. A further four doses were given throughout the next two days. Roper *et al.* (1985) state that good communication with nurses is a principal factor in the psychological element of pain relief. It is difficult to spend a lot of time with patients on a busy surgical ward, but however little time there is to spare, the quality of communication is important.

Eating and drinking

Problem Inability to eat and drink independently because of physical weakness and lack of motivation after a major operation.

Setting goals The long-term goals were for Margaret to regain independence, to obtain adequate nutrition and hydration, and for her bowel to be kept free of gastric secretions until bowel sounds were heard. Short-term goals described the steps that would need to be taken during the period in which she was dependent. Goals were set as follows: her total 24-hour fluid intake was to be 2000 ml; she was to be able to tolerate sips of water by the third day after operation, free fluids by the fifth day and small portions of food of her own choice by the sixth day; her mouth was to feel clean and moist; and she was to understand the reasons for this regime and the effect of diet on wound healing and stoma function.

Nursing actions and evaluation The rate and site of infusion were checked with other observations. Drainage from the nasogastric tube was recorded and the security and position of tube were checked. Oral hygiene was continued as often as needed. After bowel sounds were heard by the doctors on her third post-operative day she was offered sips of water hourly, increased to 30 ml hourly the next day, after her nasogastric tube had been removed. On her fifth post-operative day oral intake was increased to 50 ml hourly, and to free fluids after 8 hours as there was no vomiting. The infusion rate was changed to 500 ml per 8 hours on the fourth day and discontinued on the morning of the fifth day. A light diet was commenced the next day.

Although Margaret was pleased to 'feel more normal' her appetite was slow to return and she had little interest in food. She did not express anxieties about the effect of food on stoma function, but it seemed possible that her reluctance to eat might be associated with fear of uncontrollable flatus and ostomy output. This was discussed somewhat tentatively and she was advised to avoid spicy food or any which usually affected her in this way. She was reassured that she would be able to experiment with different foods until she had established a diet that suited her.

As it was seven days since she had eaten a high-protein diet was ordered to provide adequate nutrients in relatively small portions. Protein is necessary for wound healing and tissue repair as it forms the main part of cell structure (Tortora and Anagnostakos 1981). Any surgical procedure increases protein requirements because of increased metabolic needs for wound healing, but in addition patients with nutrient loss via wound drains or other routes have even greater needs (Hamilton-Smith 1988). Margaret was advised about continuing this diet after discharge. She was seen by the dietitian while in hospital.

Eliminating

Problem   Alteration in mode of eliminating.

Setting goals   The long-term goal was for a satisfactory pattern of elimination to be established before discharge, with a return to pre-operative independence. Short-term goals were for the colostomy to act by day 7 and to produce a soft formed stool by discharge, and for Margaret to be competent by discharge in carrying out all the steps of stoma care. A sense of competency may relieve anxiety in stressful situations and so help adaptation (Hilgarde *et al.* 1979). As she had no visual, physical or intellectual impairments it was thought that she would be able to achieve these goals in daily steps from the day her colostomy first acted. Another goal was for her to understand how to regulate her diet to suit stoma function.

For urinary elimination the goals were for the catheter to drain freely, for urine output in 24 hours to be at least 1500 ml, for Margaret to be able to pass at least 250 ml of urine within six hours of catheter removal, and for her to have no discomfort or urinary tract infection.

Nursing actions and evaluation   Minimal bleeding (not enough to measure) occurred via the stoma post-operatively. The stoma nurse visited on the first post-operative day and told Margaret that she would not touch the bag until it was necessary, to allow maximum time for healing. She visited on subsequent days to observe, and by the sixth day there was a small amount of fluid stool so the bag was changed and the stoma cleaned. The bag used was of the type that clips onto a ring on the stomahesive wafer. Margaret was shown how to do this and was able to do it herself the following day. The stomahesive wafer was changed on the ninth day after the operation and Margaret was able to do this for herself, with supervision, at the first attempt. She was reluctant to touch the stoma to wash it, although she did so without protest, showing obvious distaste at the smell. As her diet increased gradually, the stools became a little more solid and the effects of diet were discussed. Margaret was assured of continued contact with the stoma nurse after discharge and given information about skin care and the obtaining and disposing of equipment, and addresses of relevant associations. It was hoped that continued contact with the stoma nurse would encourage her to express any other anxieties she might feel, as while she was in hospital she focused only on practical aspects of the stoma.

The urethral catheter drained well and output was satisfactory. It was removed on the morning of the fourth day, after a specimen had been obtained for laboratory analysis. No urine had been passed by the end of six hours but Margaret insisted that she was not in pain and would be 'able to go later'. After nine hours her abdomen was distended, her bladder palpable and she was in obvious discomfort so she was recatheterised and 440 ml of urine was withdrawn. The catheter was left *in situ* for another 36 hours. After removal small quantities of urine between 50–70 ml were passed at each void and catheterisation in the evening showed 280 ml of residual urine. She was told that this was not unusual and that it would improve, and the reasons for the problem were explained. By her eighth post-operative day she was having no problems in passing urine and there was less than 50 ml of residual urine at the end of the day. She had reached full independence in urinary eliminating.

Problems in eliminating influence nearly all the other activities, especially eating and drinking, cleansing and dressing and expressing sexuality, so cannot be considered in isolation.

Personal cleansing and dressing

Problems Change in her physical condition would make it difficult for Margaret to carry out her usual personal hygiene activities after operation. There was a potential problem of skin damage or wound infection.

Setting goals Goals in this activity include those related to wound care as well as those related to personal hygiene and clothes. Long-term goals were for the wound to heal within twelve days with no signs of wound infection, and for Margaret to feel fresh and clean until she returned to her former independence in this activity. Short-term goals were for the wound drainage to decrease daily until

49

less than 50 ml, for the drain wound to heal within 48 hours of removal, for the abdominal wound to have no exudate or inflammation and to feel less tender by day 12, and for Margaret to take an interest in her appearance, increasing her independence at her own rate.

Nursing actions and evaluation On return from theatre the outer dressing and the drain dressing were observed for bleeding, dampness and position, with other observations. On the day after the operation the wound was cleaned with normal saline and re-dressed with an occlusive transparent dressing, then left intact until sutures were removed on the doctor's instructions on day 11, when the wound looked pink and well healed. (Occlusive dressings are also thought to relieve pain – David 1988.) Drainage was recorded daily and had decreased to 40 ml in 24 hours by day 4 when the drain was removed. The drain site looked inflamed and was not completely healed until the fifth day after removal. A wound swab was taken for identification of organisms, but no action taken as Margaret was apyrexial.

Margaret was bathed in bed on her first post-operative day and helped into a chair to allow bed-making. She continued to need help with washing in bed for the next three days but on the fifth post-operative day she walked to the bathroom for her wash. She enjoyed her first bath on the day her sutures were removed, although she left the stoma bag *in situ* during the bath because she felt anxious that it would act in the water. She was capable of self-care of the stoma now, but still found difficulty in incorporating it into her normal hygiene routine. She also seemed anxious about wearing ordinary day clothes again. Parsons (1966) suggests that in Western society, if an illness is seen to be outside the person's control, and if he has sought medical help and wants to get well, he can be excused the usual responsibilities and adopt the patient role. This role is part of the stages of illness described by Suchman (1965), the last stage being recovery and rehabilitation (Chapman 1982). It seemed that Margaret had sought medical help and thus adopted the patient role but was now not quite ready to relinquish it in this focal area of her care.

Mobilising

Problems Change in the pattern of mobilising after the operation, due to Margaret's physical condition. Potential problems of deep vein thrombosis, pulmonary embolism, chest infection and skin damage.

Setting goals The long-term goal was for Margaret to return to full independence without any complications. The steps to reach this goal included her being able to move safely with all attached apparatus, for her calves to remain of the same circumference with no tenderness, for her skin to remain intact, and for no chest pain or ·infection to develop.

Nursing actions and evaluation From the beginning Margaret was helped to change her position frequently and encouraged to carry out the deep-breathing and calf-muscle exercises she had been taught before the operation. Her calves and pressure areas were observed once per shift during the first few days and showed no signs of complications. She was shown how to get in and out of bed with the IV infusion and catheter, and started mobilising on the second day after operation, increasing at her own pace until the fifth day when she walked to the bathroom. From then on she walked around the ward freely although tiring quickly.

Working and playing

Problem The potential problem for Margaret of loneliness and anxiety about her family.

Setting goals The long-term goal was for Margaret to regain independence in work and play. Short-term goals were for her to keep in contact with her husband, family and friends; to retain some control over her own activities; to experience no isolation or boredom; and to feel her spiritual needs were being met. There is no distinct category in which to include spiritual activities, but Roper *et al.*(1985) discuss religious influence on working and playing.

Nursing actions and evaluation Visitors are welcome on the ward at any time providing they consider the well-being and dignity of all the patients. Margaret's husband visited at least once a day, and her daughters and friends were also frequent visitors. She was involved in care planning at each stage and all procedures were fully explained, so that she understood what was happening and had some control over her own care. As she was nursed in a single room it was thought that she might feel isolated, but she was quite happy about

51

this and needed no diversion other than books and visitors. Gooch (1984) feels that even short-stay surgical patients may need diversions, but Margaret was independent in this area. Communion was arranged for her on both the Sundays of her stay.

Expressing sexuality

Problem   Altered body image.

Setting goals   Helping Margaret to accept this was the long-term goal of care in this activity. The short-term goals were for Margaret to be able to make positive statements about her appearance; to touch, look at and talk about the stoma; to be able to let her husband look at it; and to be able to talk about resumption of normal activities after discharge.

Nursing actions and evaluation   Margaret was always given time, privacy and encouragement to discuss these issues. Nurses encouraged her to dress in her ordinary day clothes and to experiment with clothes which were comfortable and concealing. She was given literature about sporting activities and swimwear, and the address of a relevant local association. She was given information about controlling odour and preventing distension with flatus, and advice about diet was reinforced.

Margaret talked freely about this aspect of her life, showing concern mainly about odour, but did not mention anxieties about her sexual relationship and decided not to ask her husband to look at the stoma. He was given the opportunity to discuss aspects about which *he* felt anxious, but did not do so on any occasion. Watson (1983) claims that the post-operative period is the most crucial in terms of emotional support after stoma surgery, and patients who are allowed to explore their experience and feelings show positive improvements in self-esteem. It was difficult to evaluate how far Margaret had moved towards acceptance and it may be that her reserve was due to the temporary nature of her colostomy.

Her daughter offered to shampoo and blow-dry her hair for her during her stay, after which Margaret said that she felt 'a bit more human, at least', indicating that her self-concept had been disturbed by the alteration of her body image. Throughout her stay Margaret had not been able to – or maybe did not wish to – discuss freely this aspect of her operation, or the implications of the diagnosis. As discussed in the section on assessment, Ainslie (1981) believes that the diagnosis of cancer has of itself a detrimental effect on the body image. Margaret was almost certainly coping with feelings of loss of control of her usual body functions, which Woods and Mandetta (1975) claim affects self-concept, acceptability and perceptions of attractiveness. This problem had not been resolved by the time of discharge on May 22 but it was hoped that continued contact with the stoma nurse, in liaison with the community nurse, would help Margaret to come to terms with the anxieties she felt but could not express.

Sleeping

Problem Margaret's anxiety about an unsatisfactory sleeping pattern.

Setting goals The goal for this problem was that Margaret should be able to fall asleep within 40 minutes of settling and feel refreshed in the morning after at least six hours' undisturbed sleep. It may have been unrealistic to try to achieve undisturbed sleep in a hospital ward but being in a single room was helpful in this respect. She hoped she would be able to sleep longer once she got home.

Nursing actions and evaluation Margaret was prescribed Temazepam (20 mg) at night as required, and this dose was given every night from the third post-operative day until discharge, at her request. She said she felt much more secure if she knew she was having help to sleep and achieved a satisfactory night's sleep on most nights. She was prescribed a week's supply to take home but was advised gradually to reduce the dose as she felt more settled at home.

Dying

Problem The potential problem of Margaret and/or her family needing support in relation to the prognosis.

Nursing care and evaluation Margaret and her family were aware of the histology reports which indicated a hopeful prognosis. It was not anticipated that any further treatment such as radio- or chemo-therapy would be needed and this seemed to create an optimistic atmosphere in the family. Consequently this potential problem required no specific nursing actions other than being aware that it could have existed.

SUMMARY

On admission Margaret had adopted the patient role by seeking medical help. She had acknowledged a health problem in an AL which influenced several others, but she was still independent. The nature of the treatment altered her position on the dependence–independence continuum so that immediately after the operation she was very dependent. The goals of nursing care were designed to help her move along the continuum and to integrate into her usual activities the alterations in eliminating. Care related to discharge has been included under each activity as relevant.

EXERCISES AND ACTIVITIES

Exercise 1

Aim To apply the model's principles to the care plan.

Method Work in pairs.

Resources Care-plan documents.

Suggested time $1\frac{1}{2}$ – 2 hours.

1 List aspects of Margaret's care that are:

- common to all patients undergoing major surgery;
- common to all patients undergoing major bowel surgery;
- individual to Margaret.

2 Create a care plan for the pre- and immediately post-operative periods, based on the principles of this model. It must include the core of care which will be the same for all patients, but be flexible enough to address specific care related to different surgeons, operations and individual needs.

3 List the advantages and disadvantages of such a plan.

Exercise 2

Aim   To examine your own attitudes to altered body image and sexuality.

Method   Individual study.

Resources   Pen and paper

Suggested time   30 minutes.

1 Try to imagine that *you* have had stoma surgery and are now starting to pick up the threads of your life again. Think about how you usually carry out all your ALs and how this will change them.

2 List:
   • any changes you will have to make;
   • anxieties you may experience;
   • what support you would like, and from whom.

3 When you next nurse a patient with a stoma, reflect on whether your personal expectations have been confirmed.

Exercise 3

Aim   To consider all aspects of an altered body image.

Method   In pairs; then in a larger group discussion.

Resources   Pen and paper; flip chart.

Suggested time   1 hour for the exercise; 30 minutes for discussion.

1 In pairs:

   • List all the conditions you can think of that might affect a person's body image.
   • Select three examples from your list. Apply these to three imaginary people, making sure you have a mixture of age and gender. List the ways in which their usual ALs might be affected.

2 In a group, discuss your lists. Discussion could focus on:

   • support available in hospital and in the community;
   • the educational needs of nurses, related to this aspect of care.

Figure 4.1

PATIENT ASSESSMENT FORM	Biographical and health

Date of admission 05/05
Date of assessment 05/05   *Signature* K Evans

Patient
Surname WELLS   Forename(s) MARGARET
~~Male~~   Age 53   Prefers to be
Female   DOB 04/07/37   addressed as MARGARET

Usual address   14 Dean Road, Charbridge

Type of accommodation
   Semi-detached house

Others at this residence   Husband, daughter

Next of kin
Name   Peter Wells   Relationship Husband
Address   As above
         Telephone number Charbridge 342356

Significant others   Daughter, mother, brother, friends

Occupation   Dental receptionist

Religious beliefs   Church-goer: C. of E.
and practices   Takes communion

Recent significant
life crises   Onset of illness

Patient's perception   Good up till now.
of current health   Knows she has cancer of the bowel.

Family's perception   She hasn't seemed well for a few weeks.
of current health   They know she has cancer.

Medical information
   Childhood illnesses; tonsillectomy as child. 2 normal
   pregnancies. No other illnesses, no regular medication.
   Allergic to elastoplast.

GP
Name   Dr Brown
Address   Redwood Health Centre
         Telephone number Charbridge 428811

Consultant Mr Gray

Discharge plans
Will need contact with stoma nurse and/or
district nurse. Will require stoma supplies prior to
discharge. Out-patient appt. for 3 weeks from
discharge.

Figure 4.2

PATIENT ASSESSMENT FORM		Assessment of ALs		
Name MHRGHRET WELLS		Date of birth 04/07/37		
Stage of care Admission		Date of assessment 05/05		
		Signature R. Evans		
Activity of living	**Usual routine**	**Problems** A : Actual P : Potential		
Maintaining a safe environment	Independent	Complications of surgery (P).		
Communicating	No speech or hearing problems. Wears reading glasses.	Anxiety about the operation and its effects (P).		
Breathing	Smokes 10 cigarettes a day.	Breathing problems after operation (P).		
Eating and drinking	Good appetite. Alcohol in moderation	Loss of appetite (A). Change in diet and fluid needs (A).		
Eliminating	Altered bowel pattern. Diarrhoea, constipation. Blood in stools. Urinary: no problems.	Change in mode of eliminating with colostomy (P).		
Personal cleansing and dressing	Fully independent.	Will need help with washing post-op (A). Wound infection, skin damage post-op (P).		
Controlling body temperature	Fully independent.			
Mobilising	Fully independent.	Complications of bedrest (P).		
Working and playing	Works part-time. Dramatics, church, social outings.	Anxiety about being away from home, work and family. Isolation (P).		
Expressing sexuality	Smart appearance. Menopause at 51.	Effects of altered body image (A).		
Sleeping	Usually about 8 hours per night.	Seems anxious about sleeping pattern (A).		
Dying		May need support; also family (P).		

Figure 4.3

NURSING CARE PLAN related to ALs	
Name MARGARET WELLS	**Date of birth** 04/07/37
Stage of care Pre-op	**Date** 5th May **Signature** R. Evans

AL COMMUNICATING   **DR**

Problem(s) Possible anxiety about operation and effects

Long-term goal(s) To identify anxieties in order to relieve them.

Goal	Actions	Evaluation
Margaret to be able to express her feelings by day of op.	Allow time and privacy to listen and show interest in Margaret. Encourage discussion. R.E.	S/S Able to discuss information in own words, seems to understand well. R.E.
To show understanding about pre- and post-op. care, nature of and reasons for operation.	Explain purpose of: pre-op. diet and bowel regime, visits of stoma nurse, physio, anaesthetist. Check understanding R.E	

Figure 4.3 (continued)

NURSING CARE PLAN related to ALs	
Name MARGARET WELLS	Date of birth 04107137
Stage of care Pre-op	Date 5th May
	Signature R. Evans

AL EATING AND DRINKING; ELIMINATING	DR

Problem(s)

Long-term goal(s) Stomach and bowel to be empty by time of operation.

Goal	Actions	Evaluation
Result from colonic lavage to be clear by 8/5.	6/5 Nourishing fluids only for 2 days. 8/5 Clear fluids only. Paxolax 10mg 08.00, 14.00. Colonic lavage x2 early evening. Repeat if not clear result. 9/5 Nil by mouth after 05.00.	8/5 19.00 Clear fluid result from 2nd lavage. M.C.
Margaret to understand reasons for preparation.	Explain process of food through system reasons for needing empty stomach and bowel. R.E.	8/5 Margaret said she understood reasons but very upset in general. M.C.

59

Figure 4.3 (continued)

NURSING CARE PLAN related to ALs		
Name MARGARET WELLS		Date of birth 04/07/37
Stage of care Pre - Op		Date 5th May Signature R. Evans

AL MAINTAINING A SAFE ENVIRONMENT   **DR**

Problem(s) Lack of independence, skill and knowledge.
Potential complications of surgery.

Long-term goal(s)
　　　　To be safe in theatre and post-op period.

Goal	Actions	Evaluation
Skin to be as clean as possible.	8/5 Shave area. 9/5 Bath, dress in gown. BM.	
Any clinical abnormalities to be identified and treated.	Repeat baseline obs. TPR. BP Urinalysis.	T 36°C P82 R18. BP 135/85 (see chart). Urinalysis NAD. R.E.
Margaret to know (how to do and reason for) leg/breathing exercises before operation.	Reinforce physio's explanation. Check understanding. Tell her she will be helped post-op.	8/5 Demonstrated she could carry out exercises. Realised importance. R.E.
Safe arrival in theatre.	CHECK: Consent form Signed; no make-up or jewellery; identity bracelet on; correct x-rays and notes ready; bladder has been emptied.	All checks completed satisfactorily. R.E.
	CHECK: Give and record pre-med. Explain effects of pre-med. Leave call bell in reach.	Pre-med. given at 10.15. Asked to remain in bed. R.E.

60

Figure 4.4

PATIENT ASSESSMENT FORM		Assessment of ALs	
Name MARGARET WELLS		Date of birth 04/07/37	
Stage of care Post-op		Date of assessment 09/05	
		Signature R. Evans	
Activities of living	**Problems**		
	Actual	Potential	
Maintaining a safe environment	Dependent for safety on others.	Complications of surgery, bed rest and self injury.	
Communicating	Abdominal pain after operation.	Lack of rest. Distress.	
Breathing	Has given up smoking while in hospital.	Chest infection.	
Eating and drinking	Alteration in mode of eating and drinking.	Lack of nutrients for wound healing. Ill-effects on stoma function.	
Eliminating	Changed mode of eliminating. Dependent for care of stoma and catheter. Anxiety.	Urinary infection. Urinary retention. Stoma prolapse or retraction.	
Personal cleansing and dressing	Dependent for personal hygiene, care of wounds.	Wound infection. Skin damage.	
Controlling body temperature			
Mobilising	Unable to move freely due to physical weakness and constraints of treatment.	Deep vein thrombosis. Pulmonary embolism.	
Working and playing	Change in normal pattern of activities.	Loneliness. Boredom. Anxiety.	
Expressing sexuality	Altered body image; changed appearance and function; loss of control.	Inability to adapt to altered body image. Loss of self-esteem/perception of lessened attractiveness.	
Sleeping	Anxious about sleep pattern.	Lack of sleep, due to new environment.	
Dying	Has not expressed any feelings about diagnosis of cancer.	Anxiety about prognosis.	

Figure 4.5

NURSING CARE PLAN related to ALs	
Name MARGARET WELLS	Date of birth 04/07/37
Stage of care Post-op	Date 9th May Signature R. Evans

AL MAINTAINING A SAFE ENVIRONMENT   **DR**

Problem(s) Unable to maintain safe environment due to physical condition, lack of skill, knowledge. Potential
Long-term goal(s) haemorrhage and shock.
      Safety to be maintained while dependent.

Goal	Actions	Evaluation
Within 1 hour of return to ward: pulse rate and BP to move towards baseline.	Observations half-hourly till goal reached.	14.00 P66 BP 120/7. Outer dressing in situ, dry. BM 15.00 P76 BP 126/74. BM
Within 6 hours of return to ward: Pulse to be 80-8; BP to be 125/75 – 135/85.	Observations hourly till goals reached. Obs. 4 hrly till within normal limits for 48 hrs. Then BD.	19.00 P88 BP 130/78 T 37.6°C. TP.
Skin to be pink and warm to touch. No blood to be seen on outer dressing.	Observe lips, extremities, general appearance, outer dressing, drains, with other obs.	19.00 Colour remained good. Wound dressing in situ and dry. Drain wound redressed. TP.

Figure 4.5 (continued)

NURSING CARE PLAN related to ALs	
Name MARGARET WELLS	**Date of birth** 04/07/37
Stage of care Post-op	**Date** 9th May **Signature** R. Evans

AL COMMUNICATING	**DR**

Problem(s) Post-op. abdominal pain and nausea.

Long-term goal(s) Pain to be relieved to allow rest / recuperation.

Goal	Actions	Evaluation
Margaret to feel pain is relieved within 20 mins of post-op analgesia/anti-emetic. To ask for relief before pain is severe.	Check/clarify effects of medication with Margaret. Leave call bell within reach.	9/5 23.00 Pain relieved within 20-25 mins. of injections. Able to rest. Required analgesia 4-6 hrly. No nausea/vomiting. <center>R.P.</center>
To be comfortable during nursing care.	Change position after analgesia. Check position for comfort.	No distress caused by nursing actions. <center>R.P.</center>

Figure 4.5 (continued)

NURSING CARE PLAN	related to ALs	

Name MARGARET WELLS | **Date of birth** 04|07|37

Stage of care Post-op | **Date** 9th May
| **Signature** R. Evans

AL EATING AND DRINKING | | **DR**

Problem(s) Alteration in eating and drinking. Intravenous infusion

Long-term goal(s) Adequate fluids and nutrition while unable to eat/drink independently.

Goal	Actions	Evaluation
Bowel to be free of gastric secretions. Fluid intake in 24 hrs to be 200 ml.	At each patient contact: check IVI rate, patency and site; check naso-gastric tube is in situ, secure and draining.	9/5 IVI running at 500 ml in 6hrs. Site comfortable, no soreness. NG tube draining. T.P.
To be able to tolerate sips of water by day 3; free fluids by day 5; small diet by day 6.	12/5 Sips of water given hrly. R.E 13/5 30ml water hrly. R.E 14/5 50ml water hrly. R.E 17.00 Free fluids given 15/5 Small diet given R.E	Regime tolerated. No vomiting. IVI to run at 500ml. R.E IVI discontinued. R.E Small amount only taken. No appetite. R.E
Mouth to feel clean and moist.	Mouthwashes PRN. Lips moistened.	14/5 Dry mouth helped by mouthwashes. Vaseline to lips. R.E
To receive adequate protein for wound healing. To understand about diet and its effects on healing stoma function.	17/5 High protein diet started. Reason explained. Advised to avoid spicy food, to experiment with fruit and veg. BM.	19/5 Margaret understands need for extra protein. Appetite still poor. BM. 20/5 Weight: 9 st 3lb. M.C

Figure 4.5 (continued)

NURSING CARE PLAN	related to ALs

Name MARGARET WELLS	Date of birth 04107137
Stage of care Post-op	Date 4th May Signature R. Evans

AL ELIMINATING	DR

Problem(s) Altered mode of eliminating.

Long-term goal(s) Pattern of eliminating to be satisfactory for Margaret. To adapt to new skills for independence.

Goal	Actions	Evaluation
Colostomy to act by day 7. Soft formed stool daily by discharge. Stoma to look pink and healthy. No prolapse or retraction.	Observe stoma per shift or if uncomfortable. Check bag is secure. Advise re diet.	15/5 Fluid stool. Bag changed, stoma satisfactory. R.E. 18/5 Semi-formed stool x 2. R.E 20/5 Semi-formed stool 1 or 2x daily. M.C.
By discharge, Margaret to be able to: remove and clip on bag; change stomahesive wafer; wash stoma and skin around; understand care of skin, and dispose of soiled bags.	15/5 Nurse to do colostomy care; explain details of continuing stoma care. R.E. 16/5 Margaret to clip bag on and off. M.C. 19/5 Margaret to change stomahesive, complete stoma care. R.E.	Margaret watched without comment. R.C. 19/5 Able to manage bag and stomahesive on/off. Reluctant to touch stoma or wash as part of routine yy

65

Figure 4.5 (continued)

NURSING CARE PLAN related to ALs	
Name MARGARET WELLS	**Date of birth** 04/07/37
Stage of care Post-op	**Date** 9th May **Signature** R. Evans

AL ELIMINATING: URINARY   **DR**

Problem(s)

Long-term goal(s)

Goal	Actions	Evaluation
No discomfort or signs of infection Catheter to drain freely.	Check catheter is secure, not kinked. Observe catheter site per shift. Clean during regular washing.	10/5 Draining well. No signs of infection. R.E
Urine output in 24 hrs to be at least 1500ml.	Record intake/output.	13/5 Output satisfactory (see fluid charts) R.E
To pass at least 250ml within 6 hrs of catheter removal.	13/5 Catheter removed. Specimen to lab. R.E.	16.00 No urine passed. Catheter replaced. 440 ml withdrawn. Catheter left in situ. R.E
	15/5 Catheter removed at 07.00 Margaret reassured that problems were not unusual and explanations given. R.E	19.00 250ml urine passed in small amounts in 12 hours. Residual urine 280ml. R.E
		17/5 Passing urine freely. Output 1700ml in 24 hrs. B.H.

66

Figure 4.5 (continued)

NURSING CARE PLAN related to ALs	
Name MARGARET WELLS	Date of birth O4/07/37
Stage of care Post-op	Date 9th May Signature R.Evans

AL PERSONAL CLEANSING AND DRESSING **DR**

Problem(s) Temporary lack of independence in personal cleansing/
dressing. Potential wound infection and skin damage.
Long-term goal(s) Margaret to feel fresh, clean and attractive
while depending on others and to regain usual independence.
Wound to heal without infection within 12 days.

Goal	Actions	Evaluation
Wounds to have no exudate, redness, swelling, or continued tenderness.	Day 1 Remove dressing, clean with normal saline. Cover with op.-site strip; leave intact till suture removal. Observe daily.	10/5 Wound clean, no exudate. R.E 21/5 Wound clean, well healed. Sutures removed. M.C.
Drainage to decrease daily to under 50ml in 24hrs. Drain site to heal within 48 hrs of drain removal.	Drain wound. Measure drainage daily; re-dress with gauze dressing. 16/5 Swab from drain site to lab. M.C.	10/5 Drainage 150ml. R.E 12/5 Drainage 85 ml. Drain shortened. R.E 14/5 Drainage 45 ml. Drain removed. R.E 16/5 Drain site red and tender. M.C. 19/5 Drain site clean and healed. BM
Margaret to feel fresh and clean. To increase self-care at own rate.	Post-op. wash face and hands, clean teeth, mouth wash. Day 1: Bed bath. Day 2 Onwards: Wash in bed with help. Increase self-care as able. Encouraged to wear day clothes R.E 21/5 To have a bath. M.C.	13/5 Needs some help with washing. R.E 14/5 Washed in bathroom. Not happy about day clothes. R.E 21/5 Bathed but did not wash stoma. M.C.

67

Figure 4.5 (continued)

NURSING CARE PLAN related to ALs		
Name MARGARET WELLS		**Date of birth** 04/07/37
Stage of care Post-op		**Date** 9th May **Signature** R. Evans
AL MOBILISING		**DR**

Problem(s) Change in dependence in mobilising. Potential problems of deep vein thrombosis, pulmonary embolism, chest infection and skin damage.
Long-term goal(s) Margaret to return to full independence without complications.

Goal	Actions	Evaluation
To be able to move safely with apparatus attached.	Show Margaret how to get in/out of bed with IVI and catheter. Check ability.	13/5 Able to move with care. R.E.
Calves to remain same circumference, no redness, tenderness. No chest pain, respirations to be within 10-20 per min. Skin to be intact with no discoloration.	Observe calves and pressure areas per shift. Check all exercises are done and position changed 4 hrly.	10/5 No signs of DVT or breathing problems. Skin intact. Very good about doing exercises. R.E. 17/5 No sign of complications fully mobile. BH

68

Figure 4.5 (continued)

NURSING CARE PLAN related to ALs	
Name MARGARET WELLS	Date of birth 04 l 07 l 37
Stage of care Post-op	Date 5th May Signature R. Evans
AL WORKING AND PLAYING	DR

Problem(s) Potential loneliness and anxiety about separation from family.

Long-term goal(s) To regain independence in working and playing.

Goal	Actions	Evaluation
To keep up contact with husband, family, friends.	Visitors welcomed at any time to fit in with Margaret's activities.	Frequent regular visitors. R.E.
To retain some control over own life.	Involve Margaret in planning her care. Consider her opinions.	Showed good understanding of reasons for care. R.E
No boredom or sense of isolation.	Check whether diversions would be welcome.	No diversions required. Read a lot. R.E
Spiritual needs to be met.	Ask chaplain to visit.	Communion given x 2. R.E

Figure 4.5 (continued)

NURSING CARE PLAN related to ALs	
Name MARGARET WELLS	**Date of birth** 04 07 37
Stage of care Post-op	**Date** 15th May **Signature** R. Evans

AL EXPRESSING SEXUALITY	**DR**

Problem(s) Altered body image.

Long-term goal(s) To retain or regain good feelings about herself and her appearance.

Goal	Actions	Evaluation
To talk and act positively about appearance by discharge.	Encourage to discuss and experiment with clothes for comfort and appearance. Provide leaflets on swim- and sports-wear.	19/05 Dressed for 1st time. Feels she looks awful but better after hair done by daughter. BM. 19/05 Anxious about odour. Dislikes touching stoma but can self-care adequately. BM
To let husband look at stoma.	(No plan made for this.)	Does not see need for husband to see stoma. R.E.
To discuss resumption of normal activities.	Allow time. Ensure privacy. Encourage discussions. Involve husband. Assure of continued contact with stoma nurse. Give information of relevant associations.	Anxious about work, swimming — mainly re odour and leaking. No other worries expressed by either. R.E.

Figure 4.5 (continued)

NURSING CARE PLAN	related to ALs	
Name MARGARET WELLS	Date of birth 04107137	
Stage of care Post-op	Date 12th May Signature R. Evans	
AL SLEEPING		DR

Problem(s) Is anxious about unsatisfactory sleep pattern.

Long-term goal(s) Margaret to feel she has slept well.

Goal	Actions	Evaluation
To fall asleep within 40 mins of settling. To have at least 6 hours' undisturbed sleep To feel refreshed on waking.	12/5 Offer night sedation as prescribed after settling for night. R.E 14/5 Offer sedation after bedtime drink. Ensure position and temperature are comfortable, room is dark and quiet. Check she is sleeping. R.E.	Margaret felt secure knowing that she could have sleeping tablets. Advised to reduce them gradually after discharge. R.E

CHAPTER FIVE

Care study: a patient with a myocardial infarction

In this care study the model is used to identify problems in caring for, and to plan, implement and evaluate the nursing care given to, a patient following a myocardial infarction, from the time of admission to the time of discharge ten days later. It demonstrates the use of secondary sources of assessment information, such as that obtained from the patient's wife, and the collection of data over a period of time to suit individual circumstances. It also illustrates the relationship between medically-prescriptive and nurse-initiated care: much nursing care is based on the regime prescribed by medical staff but is modified by liaison between nurses and doctors according to individual patient progress. Medical treatment and investigations are mentioned but not described in detail. All stages of the patient's nursing care are described in the text and by means of a care plan.

The setting for this study is an acute medical ward of the Nightingale design. Primary nursing has recently been introduced and is still very much in the 'teething trouble' stage, although all the nurses are enthusiastic and committed to this method of organisation.

MR JAMES MATTHEWS

History prior to admission to ward

The patient, James Matthews, a 57-year-old Church of England clergyman, was admitted via the Accident and Emergency department (A&E) at 10.30, accompanied by his wife. He had returned to the vicarage for breakfast after morning prayers at about 08.45 and then collapsed with severe chest pains, radiating to his neck, jaw and arms. His wife called an ambulance at once. In A&E an electrocardiogram and early results of one of the blood-enzyme diagnostic tests had confirmed the presence of a myocardial infarction. Later results were able to confirm more specifically that Mr Matthews had suffered an anterior wall infarct. 1 ml Cyclomorph 15 (morphine tartrate 15 mg and cyclizine tartrate 50 mg) had been given in A&E to relieve the pain and nausea. Anticoagulant therapy had been commenced with intravenous infusion of streptokinase, 100 000 units per hour in sodium chloride, over 24 hours. This regime is followed by intravenous heparin and subsequently by oral anticoagulant therapy.

ADMISSION

The purpose of assessing activities of living is to establish the effect that the illness or treatment has upon each activity. It is necessary to know about the previous level of activities to plan care to fit in with the patient's usual patterns of living (Roper *et al.* 1985).

The staff nurse allocated to be the primary nurse for Mr Matthews introduced herself and checked that he was as comfortable as possible. She explained that she would be looking after him for the rest of his stay on the ward and outlined briefly how this would work in practice. She recognised that both patient and wife were shocked by the sudden and severe illness and decided that a full assessment would not be appropriate at this time. Mrs Matthews had acted efficiently and calmly and her presence was obviously a comfort to her husband, so the staff nurse offered her a cup of coffee and left them together for a short time. All biographical and clinical data was obtained from the medical notes. The activities of communicating, maintaining safety and breathing were considered priorities, but information related to other ALs was collected later as it was offered or observed. Primary nursing makes it more feasible to carry out only part of an assessment at a time. See Figures 5.1 (page 88) and 5.2 (page 89).

Communication

Pain and anxiety were the first priority in assessment and are included in this activity, as suggested by the model (see Chapter 3). The pain in this condition is difficult to relate logically to any specific activity of living as severe pain while it lasts may pervade every activity. (Pain is communicated by the patient both verbally and non-verbally by signs such as restlessness, facial expression or sounds of distress.) Mr Matthews said that he still felt slightly nauseous but the severe pain had been relieved. Although obviously tired, he emphasised what a shock it had been to him, and that his wife had been wonderful. He seemed anxious about *her* anxiety. Anxiety and pain were identified as actual problems.

Maintaining a safe environment

Although normally a fully independent adult, there was an actual problem of being unable to maintain his own safety while Mr Matthews was acutely ill and attached to electrical equipment such as the cardiac monitor, and while he was receiving anticoagulant drugs. The potential problem of cardiac arrest was identified as this would require regular observations to detect arrhythmias should they occur. A potential problem is defined by Kratz (1979) as: 'a problem not experienced by the patient at the time of assessment but about which there are indications that a problem will arise if no action is taken'. Its identification is based on clinical standards and professional knowledge or experience, and emphasises the preventive component of nursing (Roper *et al.* 1985). In this case it is probable that the patient was aware of the possible implications, although at this time they had not been discussed.

Breathing

Previous medical history did not indicate any problem with respiratory functions. (Information from his wife subsequently revealed that he occasionally smoked cigarettes, though not on a regular basis and he was always intending to stop.) Although he had been dyspnoeic on admission to A&E he was breathing more easily when he came to the ward. There might be a risk of accumulation of secretions in the lungs during periods of bed rest, but this was not identified as a potential problem at this stage.

It did not seem necessary to carry out further assessment at this point, so as Mr Matthews was starting to sleep, Mrs Matthews was asked for any particular details about her husband that would be helpful in enabling nurses to provide individual care. She gave the following information.

Eating and drinking

Church activities and duties seemed to take precedence over regular or relaxed mealtimes and Mr Matthews was not a fussy eater or particularly interested in food, but his wife tried to make sure that he ate a well-balanced diet, low in fats and high in fibre. He had a sweet tooth and took three teaspoons of sugar in tea and coffee.

Sleeping

He was a poor sleeper and an early riser. He had been more tired than usual in the evenings lately but often could not get to sleep quickly, some nights reading for several hours. He usually had a nightcap of whisky and water.

Working and playing

Mrs Matthews considered that her husband worked too hard in the parish, always making himself available to anyone, joining in all church activities as well as being chairman of the Parochial Church Council. He carried out all home visits without the assistance of a curate, and had little time for relaxation such as concerts or long walks. Mr and Mrs Matthews had been planning a walking holiday in the near future. She thought he would want to talk to the hospital chaplain, whom he knew fairly well, and she would also arrange for another clergyman friend and mentor to visit.

A problem of change in normal work, social and spiritual activities due to admission was identified. Also Mr Matthews might need some advice about rest and relaxation on discharge.

The rest of the data related to ALs was collected over the next 48 hours from the patient and from observation.

Eliminating

Mr Matthews usually had his bowels open daily after breakfast with no problems, and usually had to pass urine once in the night. A potential problem of constipation due to reduction in exercise and the effects of analgesia was identified. There might also be embarrassment at his temporary dependence.

Personal cleansing and dressing

This activity includes assessment of skin condition. Patches of psoriasis on both elbows were observed and Mrs Matthews was asked to bring her husband's own cream to use while in hospital. The rest of his skin was clear. A score of 17 on the Norton scale indicated that Mr Matthews was not at risk of skin breakdown, but preventive care would be included (Norton *et al.* 1962). Mr Matthews looked well built, was 1.78 m (5 ft. 10 in.) tall, and thought he weighed about 12 st. (84 kg). The actual problems of needing help to apply cream to the areas of psoriasis and to carry out usual hygiene activities while being nursed in bed were identified.

Controlling body temperature

Mr Matthews's temperature on admission was 38 °C. It is usual for the white-cell count to be raised for 3–7 days after myocardial infarction (MI) so a rise in temperature may be expected (Long and Phipps 1985). Although this was not considered a problem, regular observation would be required.

Mobilising

Although usually fully independent and very active, Mr Matthews's usual pattern of mobilising would be restricted due to the prescribed bed rest, and modified during the recovery period. Potential problems of complications of bed rest were identified. Preventive, comforting and educative aspects of nursing would be required to help him cope.

Expressing sexuality

This was not discussed at the assessment stage, but was considered a potential problem as sexual activity may have to be modified following a myocardial infarction.

Dying

Oblique reference to dying ('if anything happens') was made by Mrs Matthews within the first hours of her husband's admission, and again the next morning when she asked if the fact he had survived the first 24 hours meant that he 'had a good chance'. She sent for two of their grown-up children but was unable to contact the youngest, a student, in Europe on a walking holiday. (Results of research carried out by Thompson and Cordle (1988) showed that the fears associated with myocardial infarction are particularly stressful for wives, and suggests that early nursing intervention should be aimed at supporting them.) Mr Matthews did not express any fears to nursing staff in the early period.

The identified problems are listed in the care plan (Figure 5.3, pages 90–8).

On admission Mr Matthews was assessed as being near the dependent pole of the dependence–independence continuum in the following activities, due to his condition and treatment:

- maintaining a safe environment;
- personal cleansing and dressing;
- mobilising;
- working and playing.

He was less independent than usual in:

- eliminating;
- eating and drinking;
- sleeping;
- controlling body temperature;
- communicating (pain and anxiety increase dependence, although he was able to speak).

Although this could change he was still at the independent pole of the continuum for:

- breathing.

Expressing sexuality and dying were not assessed in this way. (Movement towards the independent pole is one way of evaluating whether or not the goals are being met after nursing intervention.)

NURSING CARE

Communicating

Problem 1   Severe chest pain caused by the blocking of a coronary artery, depriving the heart muscle of adequate blood and oxygen.

Problem 2   Anxiety and distress due to pain and uncertainty about condition.

Setting goals   The long-term goal in Problem 1 was for Mr Matthews to feel that the pain had been satisfactorily relieved; that for Problem 2 was for him to feel less anxious. Short-term goals set in order to help achieve these cannot be considered separately as one is likely to influence the other. Goals were that each episode of pain should be relieved within 5–10 minutes of intravenous or sublingual analgesia; that the pain should be relieved sufficiently to allow him to rest, sleep and remain comfortable during nursing activities; that he should be able to express his feelings about his condition and show minimal signs of distress; and that he should demonstrate understanding of the causes of pain and how it might be relieved, by resting and exercising as prescribed and by reporting episodes of pain promptly. It is not always possible to set very specific goals in the area of anxiety, especially related to time spans, but they should be measurable to some degree by the patient's behaviour. At this stage of the illness it was unrealistic to set goals with the patient, so the nurse made the decisions based on experience and clinical research or norms.

Nursing actions and evaluation   Immediate nursing actions focused on relieving pain, comforting Mr Matthews's distress, and explaining the cause of the pain, the principles of analgesia and other aspects of his treatment. Mr Matthews was encouraged to ask for pain relief promptly. During the first day, two further doses of Cyclimorph 15 were given intravenously at 14.00 and 21.30. Intramuscular injections were avoided due to their possible effect on blood enzymes (Long and Phipps 1985). Mr. Matthews reported that in each episode the pain was relieved fairly rapidly. No further Cyclimorph was required during his admission and GNT (glyceryl trinitrate, 300 μg) was administered only once, on the evening of the third day, giving rapid relief.

The need for rest and for a gradual increase in mobilisation was explained and the likely progress of recovery was discussed. An illness such as this, perceived as life-threatening, may produce a maximum of stress, and support from others as well as being able to predict likely outcomes may help to reduce it (Hilgarde *et al.* 1979). Mr Matthews was told that he would have an ECG daily for the next three days, and blood tests to monitor the anticoagulant therapy. On the third day after admission health information leaflets were offered, and he and Mrs Matthews were encouraged to discuss anxieties and to ask questions as they arose. Neither had many questions at this stage but expressed relief at the recovery so far and their implicit faith in God whatever the outcome. After experiencing further pain later that evening, Mr Matthews appeared very anxious, talked about relapses, and expressed guilt feelings about his anxiety. He wanted to talk to his clergyman friend again and would ask his wife to arrange this.

The explanations and information illustrate the educative or preventing roles of the nurse; giving medication reflects her medically-prescribed role. Cultural, social and spiritual factors influenced Mr Matthews's expression of his anxiety, which he may have perceived as a lapse in faith.

Maintaining a safe environment

Problem 1 The risk of complications (arrhythmias) due to damage to heart muscle. Alterations in blood pressure.

Setting goals The long-term goal was for Mr Matthews to suffer no arrhythmia following his MI. The short-term goals, which provide a means of evaluating, were as follows: pulse, blood pressure and respirations to remain within the normal clinical range; temperature to return to the normal range by the seventh day; no signs of cyanosis, pallor, dyspnoea or clammy skin to be observed; and any changes in cardiac rhythm to be promptly identified. In this AL, as in communicating, although the long-term goals of patient and nurse were the same, they could not be set in partnership.

Nursing actions and evaluation Arrhythmias are caused by disturbances in the conduction system of the heart. The abnormal rhythm may result in ventricular fibrillation and cardiac arrest if the heart is unable to supply its own oxygen needs but normal rhythm may be re-established if arrhythmias are promptly detected (Tortora and Anagnostakos 1981). This provides the rationale for regular clinical observations, which are the focus of nursing care.

For the first two hours after admission, pulse, respirations and blood pressure were recorded hourly; then two-hourly for the next four hours; and, as they remained within the normal range, four-hourly until the sixth day. Temperature was recorded four-hourly from the start; it reduced to 36.8 °C by the morning of the third day, peaking to 37.6 °C later the same evening. The reason for the cardiac monitor was explained to Mr and Mrs Matthews, and was observed during each patient contact. The nurse's role in this potential problem is preventive but medically-initiated, making use of observing skills. This illustrates the collaborative role of the nurse described by McFarlane (1980).

Problem 2   Lack of knowledge about precautions required while taking anticoagulant drugs.

Setting goals   The long-term goal is that Mr Matthews will experience no complications of anticoagulant therapy and will understand sufficiently to take necessary precautions. In this case the short-term goals are related to awareness of the side-effects of anticoagulant therapy so that if these occur they will be recognised promptly and appropriate action taken.

Nursing actions and evaluation   The nursing care here was mainly preventive, arising as a direct result of medical prescription. The action of anticoagulant therapy was explained and the possibility of bleeding, haematuria and petechiae identified. Mr Matthews's urine was tested daily and no haematuria observed. This was explained to Mr Matthews. As he would be continuing with oral anticoagulants, he was advised always to carry his anticoagulant card after discharge, he was told about the frequency of blood tests and where and when to attend, and he was instructed to avoid aspirin while taking these drugs. He showed a quick understanding and interest in all the information given.

Eating and drinking

Problem 1   Potential problem of fluid imbalance. Ventricular failure is a possible complication in this type of myocardial infarction.

Setting goals   The goals were that the fluid balance be maintained, with a urine output of at least one litre in 24 hours; that no sacral or ankle oedema occurred; and that Mr Matthews understood the reasons for restrictions.

Nursing actions and evaluation   The infusion was observed hourly for patency and rate, and the site observed at least four-hourly. The fluid balance was recorded for four days and the fluid intake adjusted daily according to the previous 24-hour output.

Mr Matthews's ankles and sacrum were observed for oedema four-hourly during the first three days, and subsequently once per shift. No oedema developed and his urine output remained satisfactory. The reasons for restrictions and observations were explained to him.

Problem 2   Mr Matthews was unfamiliar with dietary requirements after a myocardial infarction.

Setting goals   The major goal in this activity was for the patient (and his family) to understand the reasons for changes in diet, to know which foods to include and which to avoid, and to be aware of the importance of weight control.

Nursing actions and evaluation   Mr and Mrs Matthews were seen by the dietitian, who explained the rationale for a high-fibre, low-cholesterol diet and the need for a low sodium intake. She also provided Mr Matthews with a diet sheet for guidance although their present diet seemed fairly suitable. The primary nurse checked that they both understood all the instructions and Mrs Matthews mentioned recent articles about the efficacy of including oily fish in the diet to help to prevent further heart attacks. (Recent research reports have now confirmed this: see Burr *et al.* 1989.) Neither of them thought there would have to be very drastic changes.

Mr Matthews's weight on the fifth day was 85 kg (about 12 st. 2 lb.), so the dietitian felt there was no need to lose weight.

Eliminating

Problems   Possible constipation due to lack of exercise and effects of analgesia. Embarrassment at enforced dependence.

Setting goals   The goals set in this problem were related to the usual ways Mr Matthews had carried out this activity; thus one goal was for him to have a bowel action every day, as that was his usual pattern. Other goals were for him to be able to have his bowels open without straining, in order to avoid unnecessary effort, and for him to show minimal embarrassment during eliminating activities.

Nursing actions and evaluation　Nursing actions focused on preserving comfort, dignity and privacy and preventing further damage. Mr Matthews was prescribed Lactulose 15 ml BD (twice daily) as a stool softener. This had a good effect and after the second day he had a daily bowel action. Although still on bed rest, he was unable to use a bedpan in bed, and was lifted onto a commode by the bed. Though a fastidious man, he recognised the need to conserve his effort and accepted help from nursing staff graciously, until he was able to walk out to the lavatory on his seventh day. He had no urinary problems during his stay.

Personal cleansing and dressing

Problem　Difficulties with washing and dressing due to cardiac monitor, intravenous infusion, bed rest and general ill condition.

Setting goals　The goals in this activity were entirely patient-centred, although when a patient is this ill the nurse takes on a maternal role for a time instead of sharing the decision-making. The goals were for Mr Matthews to feel comfortable and clean with minimal effort or embarrassment.

Nursing actions and evaluation　For the first three days he was given a bed bath and was shaved by the nurse. He wore his own pyjamas, and his own prescribed cream was applied to the areas of psoriasis, which showed no changes. Mr Matthews had all his own teeth and required no help with oral hygiene other than provision of mouth-washes. From the fourth day he washed himself in bed, shaved himself and applied his cream. He said he was glad to be able to shave properly again, but was surprised at how much effort it required. On the eighth day he was able to take a bath, a cause for much celebration.

Mobilising

Problems　A change in the usual mobilising patterns, in order to rest the heart. Potential complications of bed rest.

Setting goals　The long-term goal was for Mr Matthews to be able to return to his usual level of activity without complications or further damage to the heart: this was shared by the nurse and the patient.

The time span within which this might be expected was based on the patient's condition and the nurse's experience. (Patients may be unaware of possible complications so explanations are needed even before goals are set, in order that the care can be agreed.) In this case short-term goals were for no signs of deep vein thrombosis to develop, for pressure-area skin to stay intact, and for Mr Matthews to understand the mobilising regime in order to cope with it.

Nursing actions and evaluation   The primary nurse explained that if he progressed as anticipated he would be nursed in bed completely for three days, sit in an armchair at the bedside for increasing periods for the next three days, walk to the lavatory on the seventh day, be able to take a bath with supervision on the eighth day, return to usual mobilising by the ninth day and go home on the tenth day. She explained that this regime was only a guideline and would be modified according to how he felt; she encouraged him to report promptly any pain or discomfort related to activity. He was encouraged to move around gently in the bed, changing his position at least 2–3-hourly, and was shown how to do calf-muscle exercises to aid the flow of venous blood, to help prevent deep vein thrombosis. This would also help to prevent skin damage, although assessment had not shown him to be at special risk. At times he was impatient to get going after his imposed rest; at others he felt so lethargic that he was glad to comply with the regime. He was apprehensive about further pain, and discussed ways of avoiding it.

Working and playing

Problem   Admission to hospital had caused a change in the usual routine and Mr Matthews might need to modify his lifestyle after discharge.

Setting goals   Spiritual activities are not clearly addressed in the model: they are included in the AL of working and playing. The goals were that Mr Matthews's spiritual needs would be met and that his usual family relationships would be maintained while in hospital.

Goal-setting related to modification of lifestyle requires a balance between the patient's own wishes and the nurse's knowledge. For example the nurse will be aware that even in the absence of any other factors cigarette smoking has been proved a risk factor in coronary heart disease (National Audit Office 1989), but the patient may be

83

reluctant to give up this pleasure. This was not the case with Mr Matthews, who readily agreed to try to give up smoking. Although stress is as yet an unproven risk factor, this too was discussed and the goals set with Mr and Mrs Matthews were that he would not shorten his prescribed period of convalescence, that he would utilise the services of willing lay members to a greater extent in parish affairs, and that he would try to make time for regular periods of relaxation. The couple were also given the address of the nearest branch of the Chest, Heart and Stroke Association (CHSA) as a contact point for support.

Nursing actions and evaluation   Wilson Barnett (1988) asserts that as an interactive approach has been shown to help patients cope, a mixture of teaching and counselling strategies is needed to facilitate long-term adaptation after an illness such as this. She suggests that most patients need information, reassurance and opportunities to discuss feelings, and that needs must be explored so that information may be tailored to the individual.

The primary nurse arranged for Mr Matthews to see the chaplain as soon as possible after admission and ensured that he had as much privacy as possible during visits. He asked to join other patients for communion when able, so this also was arranged. Nursing actions related to changes in lifestyle consisted of discussion and suggestions based on the information leaflets, existing knowledge, and the couple's own needs.

Mrs Matthews was included in her husband's care as much as she desired, and he was pleased to be visited by his daughter and older son and to feel that his wife was being supported. A feeling of usefulness has been identified as a need of the wives of patients after myocardial infarction (Thompson and Cordle 1988), and this did seem to help Mrs Matthews.

Evaluation in the short term would be to measure the extent to which Mr Matthews was able to carry out the modifications after discharge, and the perceived benefit. The community nurse attached to his own doctor's practice was contacted for continuing support after discharge.

Expressing sexuality

Problem   Lack of knowledge and possible anxiety about the effects of sexual activity on cardiac function.

Setting goals This was not a problem that lent itself readily to care planning in the usual manner and was not documented. The only goal was that Mr and Mrs Matthews received as much information as they required and felt confident about this aspect of their lives.

Nursing actions and evaluation The primary nurse and Mr Matthews discussed the information leaflets and resumption of usual activities after a heart attack, but it was Mrs Matthews who introduced the subject of intercourse as she felt she needed to know the risks and 'danger signs' to look for. The primary nurse suggested that abstinence was advised for four to six weeks, after which normal common sense would dictate how her husband felt about it. She suggested a few guidelines, which Mrs Matthews found useful to discuss with her husband. (Hannah *et al.* (1989) suggest that patients are often not given enough information about the resumption of sexual relations after a heart attack and recommend that in some cases specialist help may be required.)

Sleeping

Temazepam (20 mg) at night was prescribed on admission as Mr Matthews admitted to being a poor sleeper at home and anxiety about his condition might have exacerbated this problem in hospital. As this was effective most nights sleeping was not considered a particular problem during his stay.

Dying

According to the National Audit Office (1989) between 30 and 40 per cent of all major heart attacks prove fatal, with half the deaths occurring in the first two hours. Even without knowing these statistics, it is unlikely that any patient or relative does not consider the possibility of death in this situation. Mr Matthews held the traditional Christian attitudes to death, but face to face with his own mortality he was apprehensive: he confined the expression of his anxieties to his colleagues, however. Mrs Matthews openly asked about the probability of his death, was told honestly about the risks, and was kept informed at every stage of his illness. She needed reassurance that every new day increased his chances of survival and she became a source of strength and support for her husband and family. Thompson and Cordle (1988), in a discussion of research related to support of wives in this situation, say that the need to feel some hope is very important. It was thought that because Mrs Matthews had taken on such a supportive role, she herself would continue to need support in the weeks to come. This was discussed with her son and daughter and with the community nurse, before her husband was discharged on the tenth day after his heart attack.

SUMMARY

When Mr Matthews was admitted to the ward he was near to the dependent pole of the dependence–independence continuum in nearly all the activities of living. His position on the life span, combined with favourable physical, psychosocial, environmental, economic and political influences on his life, had allowed him to be a fully independent adult up to the time of his heart attack. The purpose of nursing care was to help him totally with the activities in which he was dependent, to help him incorporate necessary modifications into his lifestyle, to become independent again, and to help to prevent further problems.

The roles of nursing were threefold: those relating to ALs, medically prescribed care, and preventive care. Although in the 1985 version of the model the authors did not make explicit the comforting and preventing components of nursing, these may still be identified within other components. The role related to ALs is illustrated by helping with hygiene, eliminating and mobilising activities while Mr Matthews was unable to cope independently; and by the care given to reduce anxiety, to maintain family relationships, and to continue with spiritual activities. The comforting aspect in pain relief was combined with medically-prescriptive care, demonstrating nursing's collaborative role. The role in preventive care is demonstrated by the care to given to prevent complications of fluid imbalance, of bed rest, and anticoagulant therapy. It is also illustrated by the giving of information and advice related to diet, exercise, smoking and sexual relations, to help Mr Matthews cope confidently with usual activities without causing further damage. The medically-prescriptive component of care may be seen in nearly all aspects of this study, for doctors prescribed the drugs, mobility and clinical observation regime, but it was the nurses who explained and monitored the effects, who watched for pertinent signs and symptoms, and who ensured that care was carried out.

By discharge, Mr Matthews was once again a self-caring adult, but continuing anxiety coupled with modifications in many areas of his life may have made him feel more vulnerable in the immediate future.

EXERCISES AND ACTIVITIES

Exercise 1

Aim   To identify support available after a heart attack.

Method   Work in pairs for data collection, in the whole group for presentation.

Resources   Journals, photocopies, library material.

Suggested time   Data collection (according to course needs). Presentation according to group size.

1 In pairs:

- Compile a resource file of relevant research and literature relating to physical, emotional or psychosexual support for patients who have had a heart attack, and for their families.
- Find out to what extent support is available locally in your area for people who have had heart attacks, and for their families.
- List any obvious omissions or inequalities and your suggestions as to why these occur.

2 Presentation, in groups.

Exercise 2

Aim   To consider how the model addresses spiritual needs.

Method   In groups of three or four; as a whole group to report back ideas.

Resources   Pen and paper.

Suggested time   30 minutes for small-group work; time for reporting back, depending on group size.

1 In the small group, discuss how you would feel if faced with a patient in spiritual distress. How well does the model's philosophy address this issue? (One member of the group could act as scribe and spokesperson to report back ideas.)

2 In the whole group, the spokesperson from each small group reports the group's conclusions. The discussion could then widen to include any other human needs which members feel are not adequately addressed by the model.

Figure 5.1

PATIENT ASSESSMENT FORM	Biographical and health

Date of admission 05/08
Date of assessment 05/08   *Signature* LBrown.

Patient
Surname MATTHEWS   Forename(s) JAMES
Male   **Age** 58   Prefers to be
~~Female~~   **DOB** 06/03/31   addressed as   No preferences

Usual address The Vicarage, Church Lane, Charbury.

Type of accommodation
    Detached house.

Others at this residence Wife

Next of kin
Name Esther Matthews   Relationship Wife
Address
    As above   Telephone number Charbury 789718

Significant others Daughter, sons, John Scott (friend/colleague)

Occupation Clergyman

Religious beliefs C. of E. — would like chaplain to visit.
and practices

Recent significant Onset of illness.
life crises

Patient's perception Not sought on admission.
of current health

Family's perception Excellent health but seemed tired lately.
of current health

Medical information
Appendicectomy 1954. Fractured left clavicle 1972. No other
illnesses; no regular medication.

GP
Name Dr Pink,
Address The Lilacs, Green Lane, Charbury
          Telephone number Charbury 589881

Consultant Dr Green

Discharge plans
Will need continued support from community nurse. Out-
patient appt. for 6 weeks from discharge.

Figure 5.2

PATIENT ASSESSMENT FORM		Assessment of ALs		
Name JAMES MATTHEWS		Date of birth 06/03/31		
Stage of care Admission		Date of assessment 05/08 Signature L Brown		
Activity of living	Usual routine	Problems A : Actual P : Potential		
Maintaining a safe environment	Independant	Unable to maintain own safety while on cardiac monitor (A). Anticoagulants (P).		
Communicating	No speech or hearing problems. Wears reading glasses.	Severe chest pain (A). Anxious about condition (A).		
Breathing	Smokes occasional cigarettes.			
Eating and drinking	Good appetite. Alcohol in moderation.	Change in diet and fluid needs (A).		
Eliminating	Bowels open daily. Up to pass water x1 during night.	Constipation (P).		
Personal cleansing and dressing	Fully independant. Patches of psoriasis.	Will need help during bed rest (A).		
Controlling body temperature	Fully independent.	Temp. may be raised for a few days (P).		
Mobilising	Fully independant.	Will be on bed rest for 3–5 days (A).		
Working and playing	Clergyman. Busy parish. Likes music, walking.	Anxiety about being away from parish and family. May need to modify lifestyle (P).		
Expressing sexuality	No problems identified.	May need to modify sexual activities (P).		
Sleeping	Takes a long time to settle.	Anxiety may make this a problem (P).		
Dying		May need support; also family (P).		

Figure 5.3

NURSING CARE PLAN	related to ALs	
Name JAMES MATTHEWS	**Date of birth** 06/03/31	

Stage of care

Date 5/8

Signature L Brown

AL COMMUNICATING   **DR**

Problem(s) Pain caused by blocking of artery, depriving heart muscle of adequate blood and oxygen. Anxiety due to pain and uncertainty

Long-term goal(s) Mr Matthews to feel pain is satisfactorily relieved.

Goal	Actions	Evaluation
Each episode of pain to be relieved within 5-10 minutes of IV or sublingual analgesia. REVIEW PM.	Observe for non-verbal signs of pain or distress. Clarify effects of analgesia with Mr Matthews.	5/8 23.00 Cyclimorph effective. Sleeping. DC. 6/8 No analgesia required today. LB.
To feel comfortable during nursing care. To be able to sleep. REVIEW DAILY	Report to Dr. if GTN not effective within 5-10 mins.	7/8 Complained of chest pain at 22-30 — GTN given with rapid effect. DC.
To understand cause of pain and importance of requesting relief promptly. REVIEW DAILY	Explain physiology of pain after MI. Check understanding. Encourage to report any pain at once.	10/8 Has not complained of further chest pain. L.B. 14/8 Ready for discharge. No pain on activity. L.B.
6/8 Mr Matthews to be able to express his feelings about his illness. To show minimal signs of distress. REVIEW DAILY. L.B.	Encourage discussion, explain about ECGs, blood tests, the need for rest and gradual exercise. Offer health info. Leaflets on 3rd day. Check understanding.	7/8 Very distressed after wife left. ? Some spiritual distress. Anxious. Says he feels guilty. John Scott to visit tomorrow. SA. 8/8 Seems calm. No specific worries. SA. 10/8 Showing interest in illness and treatment. L.B. 14/8 Ready for discharge. No pain on activity. L.B

Figure 5.3 (continued)

NURSING CARE PLAN	related to ALs	

Name JAMES MATTHEWS   **Date of birth** 06/03/31

Stage of care   **Date** 5/8

Signature L.Brown

AL MAINTAINING A SAFE ENVIRONMENT   **DR**

Problem(s) ① Risk of complications (arrhythmias and changes in blood pressure)

Long-term goal(s) Mr Matthews to have no complications after his heart attack.

Goal	Actions	Evaluation
Pulse rate, blood pressure and respirations to stay within normal clinical range. REVIEW P.M.	11.00 Record pulse, resps. and B/P hrly for 2 hours, then 2-hrly for 4 hours. L.B.	5/8 16.00 B/P 135/85 mmHg, pulse 80 bpm, resps 18. L.B.
Temperature to return to normal range by day 7. REVIEW 11/8.	18.00 Record TPR and B/P 4-hrly until day 7 or until within normal range for 48 hours. L.B	5/8 Temp. 38°C on admission. L.B. 6/8 Pulse, resps and B/P within normal range. Continue obs. 4-hrly. L.B. 7/8 Temp 36.8°C this a.m. SA 22.00 Temp 37.6°C DC 11/8 All obs. within normal range. Continue obs. BD. L.B.
To understand reasons for close observation and monitoring by day 2. REVIEW 6/8	Explain purpose of cardiac monitor and importance of prompt detection of any problems.	4/8 Mrs M. watches monitor closely but shows no anxiety when at bedside. L.B. 5/8 No arrhythmia detected. L.B.
Variations in heart rhythm to be identified promptly.	Observe monitor at each patient contact or when passing bed.	10/8 No change. L.B.

Figure 5.3 (continued)

NURSING CARE PLAN related to ALs	
Name JAMES MATTHEWS	Date of birth 06/03/31
Stage of care	Date 5/8 Signature L.Brown
AL MAINTAINING A SAFE ENVIRONMENT	DR
Problem(s)② Lack of knowledge about precautions required when taking Long-term goal(s) anticoagulent drugs.	

Goal	Actions	Evaluation
Any haematuria, bleeding, or petechial rashes to be promptly identified in order to take action. REVIEW 6/8.	Test urine daily for blood and protein. Observe skin and gums daily for signs of bleeding and report at once.	6/8 Urine NAD. No bleeding seen. L.B. 8/8 Urine NAD. 8A 14/8 Urine NAD. L.B.
To know which signs to observe and what to do if bleeding occurs after discharge. REVIEW 9/8.	Explain effects of anticoagulent therapy. Encourage self-report of any bleeding. 12/8 Advise to carry anti-coag. card, to avoid aspirin, to watch for bleeding when home. Explain about blood tests. L.B.	9/8 Mr + Mrs Matthews show good understanding of situation. L.B. 14/8 Feels confident about coping with medications. L.B.

Figure 5.3 (continued)

NURSING CARE PLAN	related to ALs	
Name JAMES MATTHEWS	Date of birth 06/03/31	
Stage of care	Date 5/8 Signature LBrown	

AL EATING AND DRINKING   **DR**

Problem(s) ① Change in needs for fluid intake due to potential fluid imbalance.

Long-term goal(s)

Goal	Actions	Evaluation
IVI to run at prescribed rate. Site to remain free from excoriation.	Observe IVI hourly and site once per shift.	6/8 IVI continues as prescribed. Urine output 1350 ml. Total intake not to exceed 1850 ml. No oedema. L.B.
Urine output in 24 hrs to be no more than 500 ml less than intake (at least 1000 ml).	Record fluid intake/output Adjust intake daily based on last 24 hrs.	7/8 IVI discontinued. Output 1500 ml. Intake to be 2000 ml. No oedema. SA
Mr Matthews to understand and cope with restrictions.	Explain purpose of IVI and reasons for fluid restrictions. Check understanding	8/8 Output 1470 ml, intake to be 2000 ml. No oedema. Discontinue intake/output chart. Observe for oedema daily. SA.
Ankles and sacrum to remain free from oedema. Review daily (all).	Observe for oedema 4 hrly for 3 days, then review frequency.	12/8 No ankle or sacrum oedema. L.B.

Figure 5.3 (continued)

NURSING CARE PLAN	related to ALs	
Name JAMES MATTHEWS		Date of birth 06/03/31
Stage of care		Date 6/8
		Signature L Brown

AL	EATING AND DRINKING		DR

Problem(s) ② Lack of knowledge about dietary requirements after heart attack.

Long-term goal(s)

Goal	Actions	Evaluation
TO know which foods to include and which to avoid. TO understand reasons for change of diet. REVIEW BY DISCHARGE	Refer to dietitian. Reinforce advice given, encourage discussion. Help with selection of suitable meals while in hospital. Check weight.	9/8 Mr + Mrs Matthews think their diet is fairly suitable and will follow guidelines from dietitian. L.B. 9/8 Weight 85 kg. Dietitian thinks weight is satisfactory. L.B.

Figure 5.3 (continued)

NURSING CARE PLAN	related to ALs	
Name JAMES MATTHEWS	Date of birth 06/03/31	
Stage of care	Date 6/8 Signature L Brown	

AL ELIMINATING **DR**

Problem(s) Possible constipation due to reduced activity. Possible embarrassment.

Long-term goal(s)

Goal	Actions	Evaluation
To have daily bowel action without straining.	Give Lactulose as prescribed, explain effects. Record bowel actions daily.	9/8 Bowels open daily. Cannot use bed pan so helped on commode. Review 11/8 L.B.
To show minimal embarrassment.	Ensure maximum privacy.	11/8 Walked to lavatory. No problems. L.B.
Review 9/8		

95

Figure 5.3 (continued)

NURSING CARE PLAN related to ALs	
Name JAMES MATTHEWS	Date of birth 06/03/31
Stage of care	Date 6/8 Signature L Brown

AL PERSONAL CLEANSING AND DRESSING	DR

Problem(s) Unable to wash self as usual due to bed rest, monitor and IVI.
Psoriasis on elbows needs topical treatment.
Long-term goal(s)

Goal	Actions	Evaluation
To feel comfortable and clean with minimal effort or embarrassment. REVIEW 8/8.	Bed bath for 3 days. Help with shave, teeth. Give assisted wash in bed on days 4-7. May have supervised bath on 12/8.	8/8 Washed and shaved self. REVIEW 11/8. SA 11/8 Walked to lavatory for 1st time, had wash in bathroom. L.B. 12/8 Managed bath without pain. L.B
Skin lesions to show no signs of exacerbation. REVIEW 12/8	Apply Mr Matthew's own cream as prescribed.	No change in psoriasis patches. Apply own cream. Problem discontinued. L.B.

96

Figure 5.3 (continued)

NURSING CARE PLAN	related to ALs	

Name JAMES MATTHEWS   **Date of birth** 06/03/31

Stage of care

Date 6/8

Signature L Brown

AL MOBILISING   **DR**

Problem(s) Change in usual mobilising in order to rest heart muscle
Potential complications of bed rest.

Long-term goal(s)
      To return to usual level of independent activity by day 9.

Goal	Actions	Evaluation
No signs of DVT to occur. Pressure-area skin to remain intact with no discoloration. REVIEW DAILY	Teach calf-muscle exercises. Encourage him to do them and to change position 2-3 hrly. Observe calves daily for redness, tenderness or swelling; pressure areas once per shift.	7/8 Mr Matthews needs to be reminded to change position. No signs of DVT or skin damage. REVIEW 8/8 SA 8/8 Sat in chair for ½ hr. SA
Mr Matthews to understand need for rest and exercise and to be able to increase activity at own rate.	Explain regime and that it will be modified according to how he feels. Explain reasons for all care. Observe for signs of pain related to activity.	12/8 Is walking and self-caring without ill effect. L.B. Problem discontinued. L.B.

Figure 5.3 (continued)

NURSING CARE PLAN related to ALs		
Name JAMES MATTHEWS	Date of birth 06\03\31	
Stage of care	Date 7\8	
	Signature SA	
AL WORKING AND PLAYING		DR

Problem(s) Change in social, working and spiritual activities. Need to
Long-term goal(s) modify lifestyle on discharge.

Goal	Actions	Evaluation
Mr Matthews to be able to continue to worship and to maintain normal family relationships while in hospital. REVIEW 10/8.	Help family to feel welcome on ward. Include Mrs Matthews in care when possible, as desired.	7/8 Visited by son and daughter, very emotional. SA 10/8 Mrs Matthews is keen to help as much as possible. L.B.
	Ask chaplain to visit. Liaise with Mrs. Matthews for visit from Mr Scott Ensure privacy for visits.	10/8 Has been visited by chaplain and friend. Has taken communion with other patients. L.B.
To recognise need for some changes after discharge.	Encourage discussions about modifications to lifestyle with family. Arrange for community nurse to visit on discharge Inform about local Chest, Heart and Stroke Association.	12/8 Is going to stop smoking and will try to arrange extra lay help in parish. L.B.

CHAPTER SIX

Care study: a child needing eye surgery

This chapter illustrates the use of the model to assess the needs of, and to plan, implement and evaluate the nursing care for, a child undergoing elective eye surgery. Emphasis is placed on the influence of the life span on activities of living and therefore on the nursing care associated with them. The discussion focuses on pre-operative care, but all the nursing care is included in the care plan. It is the story of three-year-old George, admitted to the children's ward for correction of a squint in his right eye, and of his mother Linda, who stayed with him.

It is the practice on this ward to invite parents and children to visit the ward about a week prior to elective surgery. A maximum of four children attend any one session: during it pre-admission assessing takes place, the children are weighed and measured, and ward routine, the facilities and the sequence of events related to the operation are exlained. Parents and children see a short video about the ward, are shown round the ward, visit the theatre nurses, and are helped to become familiar with ward and hospital life in general.

GEORGE LAWRENCE

Pre-admission assessment

George was brought to the ward by his mother, Linda, an 18-year-old single parent, living with her parents and her younger sister and brother in a tied farm cottage. Linda worked part-time at the checkout at the local hypermarket and George's care was shared between her and his grandmother, who did not work outside the home. He was quiet and solemn during the interview and at one point retrieved a dummy from his mother's handbag which he sucked for the rest of the time. Linda said he chatted non-stop at home and usually only had the dummy at bedtime. Details of the assessment will be included as a basis for care planning in the text, and may be seen in Figures 6.1 (page 109) and 6.2 (page 110).

PRE-OPERATIVE CARE

George arrived on the ward clutching his tipper truck: he was accompanied by his mother and grandfather. He was shown where Linda would stay while he was in hospital. A 1988 Health Service report outlined by Sadler (1988) states that a parent staying with a child in hospital may reduce the length of stay by as much as 50 per cent: the report recommends that provision should be made for parents of all under-fives to be accommodated overnight. This reflects the findings of the well-known work by Bowlby (1973) on separation and anxiety.

George greeted the nurse quite happily and thought it was funny that her name was Debbie, the same as his young aunt. He was shown his cot and locker and helped his mother unpack his belongings before his grandfather went home.

As well as sociocultural and environmental factors, George's physical and cognitive stage of development influenced the way he carried out his activities of living and were the focus of planning. As long as thirty years ago the Platt report recommended that children should be nursed in specially designated units by nurses with paediatric qualifications, in order that their special needs were recognised and catered for (HMSO 1959). Lewer and Robertson (1983) give a clear account of development of the pre-school child and its relevance to hospital admission, which will be included as relevant in the account of his care, under the headings of individual ALs. For a diagram showing George's level of independence, see Figure 6.3.

Communication was the major focus for nursing care and influenced most other activities. The care planned for each activity is described in relation to physical, social and cognitive development, the ability to communicate and understand. Changes in environment or routine and use of unfamiliar language were identified as possible causes of anxiety. The nursing care before the operation focused on physical and emotional preparation for surgery, involving to a greater or lesser extent most of the activities of living. It also included carrying out care related to medical prescription. The children's ward did not carry out primary nursing in the strictest sense for all patients. George would be nursed with three other

Figure 6.3 *Examples of the dependence status of a child*

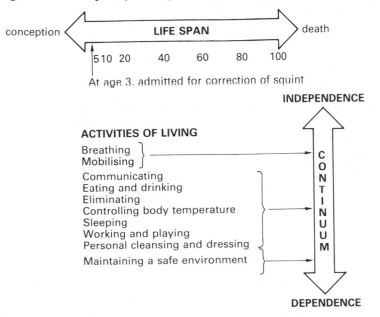

children having ophthalmic surgery, in a six-bedded bay with one nurse responsible for their care for the whole span of each shift.

Extracts from the pre-op. care plan are shown in Figure 6.4 (pages 111 and 112).

Communicating

Research showing that anxiety may be reduced by adequate information has been discussed in previous chapters. For George to understand such information the nurse needs to apply her knowledge of child development when she talks to him. Vocabulary increases to as many as 1500 words during years 2–5 so George might be expected understand plurals, know his own name, address, age and gender. Bee and Mitchell (1989) claim that children of this age understand short, simple, often-repeated sentences which refer to objects or people rather than abstract ideas. Repeating the child's response provides him with positive reinforcement (children often repeat things to themselves as a strategy for remembering what they've been told). Small children also over-extend the meanings of words – all animals may be dogs, or all women mothers. They begin

101

to understand adult roles by pretending games, such as shopkeeper and customer, or from picture books or stories (Roper *et al.* 1985). The communicating aspect of care will be related to each activity of living and is described here in relation to general information-giving.

Goals   These were for George to explain in his own words what was going to happen while he was in hospital and to show fewer signs of anxiety. These were long- and short-term goals as the information would be given in stages. Lewer and Robertson (1983) say that information should be given as short as possible a time before the event, and the sequence explained in relation to recognisable points in the child's experience, such as bedtime or dinner time.

Nursing actions and evaluation   Information was given in two stages. Although described 'compartmentally' other nursing activities were carried out concurrently.

First, when George had installed himself comfortably in his own cot area, the nurse started talking to him about his previous visit and he indicated quite happily that he remembered the toys and the weighing machine. She told him that he could play with the toys during the morning and the doctor would come to see him to say hello. George volunteered that the doctor would make his eye better and he would show him his tractor. The nurse also told him that Linda would give him a bath later on and dress him in the special clothes he'd seen when he came before. (The play component of information will be included in the AL of working and playing.)

Secondly, just before the pre-medication was due, more information was given. George and the rabbit were dressed in their gowns, both wearing wristbands with their names on and sitting on Linda's lap. (At this age children invest their toys with reality, thinking the toy perceives as they do.) George was reminded about meeting the theatre nurses and told he could have a ride on the trolley to see them and the doctor again. He was told that he would feel sleepy and the doctor would make his eye straight while he was asleep; being asleep would enable him to keep really still. He was reassured that his mother would be with him all the time till he woke up back in the ward. (Research studies have shown that children are less distressed during induction of anaesthesia if a parent is present and many anaesthetists and nurses support this practice – Dewar and Glasper 1987; Hawthorne 1974.) George repeated some of this to his rabbit and seemed contented. He settled with his dummy after his pre-med with no problems. The pre-operative checklist was completed and the 'consent to anaesthetic' form signed.

102

Although his vocabulary was increasing at this period, it would not include many of the words used familiarly by nurses. Roper *et al.* (1985) describe technical expressions used by an occupational group as their 'language culture'. It is essential that nurses use familiar words to explain care to a child, avoiding misunderstanding and added anxiety. All the care was explained to Linda.

Working and playing

It is generally accepted that playing facilitates learning and social development.

Goal George should be familiar with ward situations and able to express any feelings he cannot express verbally.

Nursing actions and evaluation Intervention in this activity illustrates the collaborative role as the nurse or play leader might take part. George and the other three children were provided with Fuzzy Felt hospital games, picture books about children in hospital, theatre gowns and caps, nurses' caps, a stethoscope and toy thermometers, among more familiar toys. They were encouraged to play freely and imaginatively, but were guided by the play leader if necessary. Questions were answered and play was observed. Roper *et al.* (1985) agree that development depends on adults encouraging play, saying that four conditions necessary for satisfactory play are toys, space, time and playmates. George was quite sociable, and seemed to enjoy the morning. He was concerned about a timid little boy who wouldn't join in, trying to include him in all activities. (Hoffman proposes that children as young as two or three may be empathic, responding to the distress of another person – Bee and Mitchell 1989.)

Maintaining a safe environment

Children aged between two and five years are becoming more adventurous and are more willing to explore without their mother. At the same time this age group has a limited concept of safety so care planning needs to include interventions to address this issue. George was nursed in a six-bedded bay with windows opposite the nurse's station so that he could be observed at all times. The children are never left alone in the immediate pre- or post-operative periods.

Nursing actions and evaluation When George was ready for his pre-med. he was told that he would be sleepy for a while and that the sides of the cot would be put up to stop him falling out and hurting himself. He described a similar accident at home in which he had bruised his knee. On his first post-op. day he managed to climb out anyway, so the side was left down thereafter.

Eating and drinking

At George's age a child is becoming independent but may need help to complete the meal. George was independent but did not want to sit at table and eat proper meals, preferring crisps, biscuits or icecream. During such a short stay this did not present a problem.

Goal The stomach should be empty before the operation to prevent inhalation of contents. Both child and mother should understand the reason for having no food or drink.

Nursing actions and evaluation The nurse decided not to discuss this aspect of care with George unless it became necessary. The concept of food in the stomach causing respiratory problems would be too difficult to understand. As all four children were in the same situation, none of them would be eating or drinking so he might not think of it himself. Bee and Mitchell (1989) claim that three-year-olds understand that cause comes before effect so this principle may be used to explain the reason for 'nil by mouth' in appropriate phraseology. However a simple statement to the effect that he would be able to eat and drink after the operation, and that all the children were in the same situation, might sustain him. This was explained to Linda, and a notice fixed to his bed.

Eliminating

George was clean and dry by day but not at night. He managed by himself in the lavatory with the exception of bottom-wiping. At three, George was at the stage described by Erikson (1950) as the stage of 'autonomy versus shame', where he was gaining independence and starting to exercise some choice but also making mistakes or experiencing the shame of failure. A change of environment might cause regression in newly-acquired skills, making him feel embarrassed and ashamed.

Goal George should maintain without embarrassment the pattern of eliminating established at home.

Nursing actions and evaluation Linda said that he was beginning to be self-conscious about wearing a night nappy and when he had settled after the operation, she was going to give him a trial run without it. He used a potty in the bathroom at home, so he was able to continue. He was encouraged to pass urine before the operation but was unable to, so a nappy was put on after he was asleep to avoid any feelings of shame or distress. He had no problems during his stay.

Controlling body temperature

Goal Temperature, pulse and respirations to remain within normal range for this age.

Nursing actions and evaluation George had never had his temperature taken but he recognised the thermometer from the play described earlier. He was quite happy to sit with it under his arm, and the rabbit was treated the same way. A child of this age is partly dependent on others in temperature control, such as clothing and ventilation. In addition the heat-regulating system is sensitive in young children and prolonged crying may raise the temperature.

POST-OPERATIVE CARE

The focus of the immediate post-operative care is to maintain a safe environment during the period when the patient is unable to do so independently; care also aims to prevent complications such as an obstructed airway or hypovolaemic shock. Later care includes helping the patient to carry out his usual activities of living in a way that causes minimal disruption to his usual routine, as well as the specific care related to the particular operation.

It is difficult to impose mobilising restrictions on young children and in this case the level of activity was set by his feeling of well-being. George made a quick recovery, demonstrated by climbing out of his cot on the morning after his operation. Thereafter, his mother took over the care related to usual living activities as she would at home, while the specific care of his eye was carried out initially by a nurse and subsequently by Linda with support and supervision.

George was discharged on the second post-operative day. His eye looked clean and Linda was given clear instructions about care of the eye, including administering ointment, and told the date of the follow-up appointment. The health visitor was asked to visit within 24 hours of discharge, to check that Linda was coping and understood all the information she had been given. This is usual practice for the under-fives. Research by Coulson (1988) showed that 68 per cent of mothers would have liked fuller or clearer explanations about the continuing care of their children on discharge.

Figure 6.5 (pages 113 and 114) shows extracts from the post-op. care plan; Figure 6.6 (pages 115 and 116) shows care related to medical prescription.

SUMMARY

Nursing knowledge is a common element of all nursing models but the emphasis on content differs according to the model philosophy. In the Roper–Logan–Tierney model the knowledge is concerned with the twelve activities of living, the factors that influence their performance, and the extent of independence in each activity. In George's case, this included knowledge of biological and psycho-social child development theories as the planning of his care focused on his developmental stage on the life span, as well as knowledge gained from work such as that done by John Bowlby on the effect of separation on young children (Bowlby 1973). The aim of nursing in this model is to keep to the patient's usual model of living as much as possible: this is even more important for a small child. Care planning also needed to include provision for George's mother, still very young herself, and used skills of communication, information-giving and teaching. Because this was a planned admission, the child and the mother were able to familiarise themselves with the ward and the staff before the admission.

EXERCISES AND ACTIVITIES

Exercise 1

Aim To identify appropriate methods of giving information to a pre-school child.

Method Collection of visual aids and play material, working individually.

Resources   Variable, according to what is planned.

Suggested time   A minimum of one clear week, but this will depend on the type of course and on other commitments.

1 Design and produce a booklet or series of cards to be used for giving information to the pre-school child coming into hospital for correction of a squint. (This could be applied to any other operation for a child, such as a tonsillectomy.)

2 List additional play materials that could supplement the visual information.

Exercise 2

Aim   To apply knowledge of child development to care planning.

Method   Work in pairs, then in groups of six.

Resources   Identified books (see below); posters.

Suggested time   A minimum of one clear week for the first activity, but this will depend on the type of course and on other commitments; 2 hours for the group work.

The model literature describes eight developmental stages similar to those proposed by Erikson in his life-span development theory. It also draws on Piaget's cognitive development theory and the work done by John Bowlby on attachment, separation and loss.

1 Each pair is allocated a theory to work on.
   • When you have found the relevant work, prepare a précis giving a clear summary of the theory to present to the rest of the group.
   • List the data which you think you would find especially helpful in planning the care of a young child in hospital.

2 In a group of six, each pair should present their summary and ideas. Pooling the information from the three works, plot a life span with identifiable stages and create an educational poster for use on a ward.

References

Bowlby, J. 1953. *Child Care and the Growth of Love*. London: Pelican.
Bee, H. and Mitchell, S. 1980. *The Developing Person : a life span approach.*

New York: Harper and Row. This book discusses the work of Erikson and Piaget: if you wish to read these authors' own words, try Erikson, E. H. 1950. *Childhood and Society* (New York: Norton) and Piaget, J. 1952. *The Origins of Intelligence in Children.*

Exercise 3

Aim   To identify ways in which children communicate.

Method   Individual observation; group discussion (6–8 members).

Resources   Children at play; pen and paper.

Suggested time   Observations over a planned period for a minimum period of 10 minutes per observation; group work 1 hour (or according to the size of the group).

1 Watch a child or group of children at play. Observe:

- what type of games they play;
- what play material they use;
- the conversations they hold and with whom or what.

Make a note of the age and sex of each child.

2 Present your findings and select a scribe to record observations under the following headings.

- age;
- sex;
- circumstance.

Discuss similarities and differences within these groups.

Figure 6.1

PATIENT ASSESSMENT FORM (child)	Biographical and health

Date of admission 21/10
Date of assessment 15/10   *Signature* S. Martin

Patient
Surname LAWRENCE   Forename(s) GEORGE ANDREW
Male   Age 3   Prefers to be
~~Female~~   DOB 03/07   addressed as GEORGE

Usual address 3 Tor Farm Cottages, Dryford-on-Char, nr. Charbridge

Type of accommodation
Terraced cottage

Others at this residence Mother, grandparents, aunt, uncle

Next of kin
Name Linda Lawrence   Relationship Mother
Address As above
     Telephone number Dryford 4326

Significant others Grandparents, aunt, uncle

Support services None

School/college/nursery None

Religion Baptist   Baptised? Yes

**Recent significant
life crises** None

Parents' perception Good. Is worried about him having an
of child's health operation.

Medical information   Immunisations All up to date.
Chickenpox 6 weeks ago. Very few colds.
No history of diabetes, no febrile convulsions.
No known allergies

GP
Name Dr Gold
Address Health Centre
     Telephone number Dryford 5871

Other   Health visitor
Name Mrs Brass
Address Health Centre
     Telephone number Dryford 5871 ext 220

Consultant Mr Silver

Discharge plans No special plans required. Mother will need to
be familiar with care of eye and process of recovery. Out-
patient appointment for 3 weeks from discharge.

Figure 6.2

PATIENT ASSESSMENT FORM (child)		Assessment of ALs	
Name GEORGE LAWRENCE		Date of birth 03/07	
Stage of care Pre-admission		Date of assessment 15/10	
Height 96 cm	Weight 15.5 kg	*Signature* G. Martin	
Activity of living	**Usual routine**	**Problems** A : Actual P : Potential	
Maintaining a safe environment	Can climb out of cot and manage stairs safely. Understands simple precautions related to hot or sharp objects.	Too young to be responsible for own safety (A). Complications of operation and anaesthetic (P).	
Communicating	No speech or hearing problems. Mother says he speaks quite well.	Very shy and quiet (A). Anxiety about new environment (P).	
Breathing	No apparent problems. Gets very few colds.		
Eating and drinking	Likes sweets, crisps, biscuits, sugar puffs, etc. Poor eater at mealtimes. Has milk in bottle at bed time.	Change of routine and effects of operation may affect appetite. (P).	
Eliminating *Words used*	Clean & dry by day. Wears nappy at night. Uses potty by self and manages own clothes but not bottom wiping. Potty. Pee. Big Poo.	Change of routine and effects of operation may cause 'accidents' or embarrassment (P).	
Personal cleansing and dressing	Undresses self and cleans own teeth but sometimes refuses. Does not dress or wash self. Dislikes washing.		
Controlling body temperature	No history of pyrexia or convulsions. George is dressed appropriately for weather.	Vulnerable to raised body temp. if upset, due to age (P).	
Mobilising	Fully independent. Walked at 11 months. Rides bike with stabilisers.		
Working and playing	Does not go to play school. No children to play with near home. Favourite toy is tipper truck. Takes soft rabbit named 'Dog' to bed.	Change of routine and environment, separation from family and pets (A). Anxiety (P).	
Expressing sexuality	Mother says he is not modest or embarrassed about undressing or lavatory. Has not commented on appearance of squint.		
Sleeping	No regular bedtime. Sleeps in cot in room with mother and her sister. No day nap. Takes bottle and dummy to bed. Sleeps about 10 hours.		
Dying			

Figure 6.4

NURSING CARE PLAN related to ALs	
Name GEORGE LAWRENCE	Date of birth 03/07 (Age 3)
Stage of care Pre-Op.	Date 21st October
	Signature P. Jones

AL MAINTAINING A SAFE ENVIRONMENT	DR

Problem(s) Unable to maintain own safety independently, due to age (A).

Long-term goal(s) To remain free from accidents or injury.

Goal	Actions	Evaluation
George will be attended at all times. Mother will be able to locate all facilities and nurse call-bell, and understand reasons for care given or any restrictions imposed. REVIEW DAILY.	Nurse to stay within sight of child whenever mother is away. Ensure cot sides are up at all times. Show round ward, and room that Linda may use.	22/10 Lively post-op. day. Mother present except for meals and is coping well. George is very active, climbing and running. No problems. P.J.

111

Figure 6.4 (continued)

NURSING CARE PLAN related to ALs	
Name GEORGE LAWRENCE	**Date of birth** 03/07 (Age 3)
Stage of care Pre-op.	**Date** 21st October
	Signature D. Jones.

AL COMMUNICATING	**DR**

Problem(s) George is quiet and shy in new environment. Linda seems very anxious about operation (A).

Long-term goal(s) George and Linda to feel confident and less anxious.

Goal	Actions	Evaluation
Linda to show understanding of operation and related care by paraphrasing all information. Linda and George to be able to make needs/worries known.	Reinforce information given prior to admission. Explain pre- and post-op. care, sequence of events, time and places related to operation. Check understanding. Explain pre- and post-op. care to George, using pictures and toys to clarify.	21/10 Linda needed further explanations about operation. Very upset when her father went home, glad to talk to other mothers. George settled well before theatre and talked at length about tractors. The rabbit has eye pad, theatre gown and nappy on. D.J.

Figure 6.5

NURSING CARE PLAN related to ALs	
Name GEORGE LAWRENCE	**Date of birth** 03\07 (Age 3)
Stage of care Post-op.	**Date** October **Signature** D. Jones

AL ELIMINATING	DR

Problem(s) Change in routine of all ALs after operation.

Long-term goal(s) All needs to be met with minimal disruption to usual ways of carrying out activities.

Goal	Actions	Evaluation
To pass urine within 8 hours of operation. To use potty as at home.	Encourage George to pass urine when properly awake.	19.00 Has passed urine AT. 22/10 Is using potty well. Problem discontinued. D.J.
To tolerate fluids and diet by day 1.	Offer sips of water when awake. Offer bottle or food from 6 hours post-op. if tolerating fluids.	22.00 Fluids taken well. Bottle given and settled back to sleep. EF 22/10 Very little diet taken. Asking for sweets and coke. No further problem.
To look clean and feel comfortable.	Sponge face and hands, change into own pyjamas when awake post-op. Encourage mother to care for him as at home with help if needed.	22/10 Linda has cared for him totally. No further problem. D.J.
To feel occupied and contented while on bed rest after operation. Mother to understand need for rest.	Keep child in bed for at least 24 hours, explain why. Check he has enough to keep him occupied.	22/10 Climbed out of cot repeatedly. Played with tipper truck under cot most of morning, became more active as day progressed. No ill-effects seen. D.J.

113

Figure 6.5 (continued)

NURSING CARE PLAN	related to ALs

Name GEORGE LAWRENCE	Date of birth 03/07 (Age 3)

Stage of care Post-op.	Date 22nd October Signature D Jones.

AL PERSONAL CLEANSING AND DRESSING.   **DR**

Problem(s) Potential wound infection in eye.

Long-term goal(s)   No wound infection to occur.

Goal	Actions	Evaluation
Wound to begin to heal by discharge with no redness, swelling or exudate from eye, or pain.	22/10 Remove pad, bathe eye with normal saline. Instil prescribed ointment and apply clean pad. Bathe eye and observe for signs of infection. BD.	Eye looks clean. Difficulties with ointment. D.J. 23/10 No signs of infection. Looks clean. Seen by Dr for discharge and continue care at home. S.M.
Temp to remain between 35.5°C and 37°C.	Record daily if within normal range.	No pyrexia. D.J.
Mother to feel confident about eye care on discharge.	Demonstrate application of ointment, supervise Linda when she applies it.	Linda finds it difficult but thinks her mother will help. D.J.

Figure 6.6

NURSING CARE PLAN related to medical prescription	
Name GEORGE LAWRENCE	Date of birth 03/07 (Age3)
Stage of care	Date 31st October
	Signature D. Jones

Problem(s) Potential complications of anaesthetic. Inhalation of
Stomach contents. (P)
Long-term goal(s)
George will experience no complications.

Goal	Actions	Evaluation
Stomach to be empty prior to operation.	Check that George has had no food or drink since 7a.m and that he has none before operation. Explain reasons.	Has had nil by mouth since 6.45 a.m.. D.J.
Mother to understand reasons for all care.	Complete pre-operative checklist with Linda. Ensure George passes urine pre-op. Explain that he must stay in cot after pre-med.	Checklist complete. Has not passed urine. Pre-Med given. D.J.
George to be separated from mother as little as possible.	Linda to accompany George and wait until he is anaesthetised.	To theatre at 14.15. D.J.

115

Figure 6.6 (continued)

NURSING CARE PLAN related to medical prescription

Name GEORGE LAWRENCE	Date of birth 03	07 (Age 3)

Stage of care	Date 31st October
	Signature D. Jones

Problem(s) Hypovolaemic shock post-operatively (P).

Long-term goal(s) No hypovolaemic shock to occur.

Goal	Actions	Evaluation
Airway to remain clear. No cyanosis or distress.	Nurse in semi-prone position. Stay with child for first hour.	15.00 Returned from theatre. Pulse 96 bpm. Condition satisfactory. Eye pad secure. R.J.
Pulse to remain between 70 and 120 bpm. Pulse to stabilise at baseline within 1 hour of return to ward.	Record pulse on return to ward. Repeat half-hrly if outside normal range.	18.00 Temp 37°C pulse 92 bpm, resps 24 per min. Awake and asking for drinks. A.J.
Temp. to be within normal range by 4 hrs post-op.	Record TPR 4 hours post-op Repeat 4 hrly for 24 hrs.	No fresh bleeding. P.J.
Skin to remain pink, warm and dry to touch.	Observe skin and eye pad hourly after first hour.	Linda happy to stay with him. R.J.
No fresh bleeding to be seen on eye pad.	Explain process of recovery and points to observe, to mother	

CHAPTER SEVEN

Care study: an elderly lady

This chapter illustrates how the model may be used in different areas for the same patient. It paints a picture of the nursing care received by an elderly lady over a period of ten weeks, in an orthopaedic trauma ward, in the community, and in an elderly care ward. Emphasis is placed on the changes in dependence. Not every aspect of the lady's care is described, but some areas are discussed in detail.

MRS ANNIE COLEMAN

At the time of admission Annie was a 78-year-old widow who had lived alone since her husband had died six years before. She had lived in the same terraced house in the centre of town for the past forty years. Two years prior to the accident that brought her to hospital she was thought to have had a transient cerebral vascular accident (CVA), which had left her with a very slight weakness in her left hand. Her only medication was bendrofluazide (2.5 mg daily) for mild hypertension, which had been diagnosed six years before.

At teatime on 11 February, she fell from a chair when changing a light bulb, but was able to drag herself along the floor to telephone a neighbour. She was admitted to the accident and emergency department (A&E) at 19.00; an X-ray confirmed that the neck of the right femur had fractured.

ADMISSION

In A&E intramuscular Pethidine (25 mg) was given for pain, prior to Annie's admission to an eight-bedded bay on the thirty-bedded orthopaedic ward. Team nursing is organised on this ward in the mornings, one team of nurses caring for all patients in one half of the ward, allocating the patients within that area.

Annie was accompanied by her neighbour, who had contacted her son. Skin traction was applied and the reasons explained. Annie said she felt reasonably comfortable, had understood what she had been told about her operation, and felt able to answer questions about herself. As she was also alert it was decided to assess her nursing needs at once. It is important to do this with discharge in mind, especially when the patient is elderly and living alone.

The ward has devised a dependence–independence scale for eight ALs, for use as an assessment and evaluation tool ('1' represents 'most independent'). This scale is used to assess usual independence, the status on admission, and the status at any other stage; scores are recorded in documents. For a guide to this scale, see Figure 7.1.

For assessment records and care plans, see Figures 7.2–4 (pages 135–43). For a comparison of dependence levels at three stages of care, see Figure 7.8 (page 154).

Figure 7.1 *Guidelines for assessing activities of living on the dependence–independence scale*

```
          ASSESSING ALS

MAINTAINING A SAFE ENVIRONMENT

1 Is able to carry out all ALs safely.
2 Is unsafe in one AL infrequently (e.g.
  bathing).
3 Is unsafe in more than one AL (e.g. walk-
  ing, bathing, or on stairs). May be
  mildly confused.
4 May be unsafe at some time in all ALs or
  very confused.
5 Needs constant supervision (e.g. is un-
  conscious, suicidal, or very young).

COMMUNICATING

1 Communicates fluently and coherently.
2 Has mild sensory deficits (e.g. deafness
  or a stammer).
3 Has profound sensory deficits (e.g. is
  totally blind or deaf).
```

118

4 Is affected by mental/intellectual factors (e.g. is very young, confused, or depressed).
5 Is unconscious or has severe learning difficulties.

BREATHING

1 Has no breathing problems.
2 Is vulnerable to infection (e.g. is a heavy smoker or post-op.).
3 Has chronic respiratory problems.
4 Is in acute respiratory distress or is unconscious.
5 Requires a respirator.

EATING AND DRINKING

1 Is totally independent or is taking nil by mouth.
2 Needs minimal help (e.g. cutting food or mopping up).
3 Needs feeding with food and drinks or has post-op. IVI or nasogastric tube or is newly diabetic.
4 Is subject to persistent vomiting or is reluctant to eat.
5 Requires total parenteral feeding or lacks a swallow reflex or is unconscious.

ELIMINATING

1 Is independent or can cope with a stoma, a catheter or incontinence aids.
2 Needs minimal or occasional help (e.g. with a commode, a bedpan or stoma care).
3 Cannot manage clothing or cleaning. Is occasionally incontinent.
4 Cannot manage a stoma or a catheter or is frequently incontinent of urine or faeces.
5 Is paralysed or unconscious or is a baby or very young or is doubly incontinent.

MOBILISING

1 Mobilises independently, perhaps using aids.
2 Walks short distances, indoors only <u>or</u> is independent but uses a wheelchair; can self–transfer.
3 Can walk with one person; may need help to transfer.
4 Has been prescribed bed rest: can move in bed; is alert and orientated.
5 Is bed– or chairfast; cannot move or turn self <u>or</u> is unable to understand the rationale.

PERSONAL CLEANING AND DRESSING

Washing and dressing
1 Is independent: may manage with aids.
2 Manages all personal care with minimal or infrequent help (e.g. needs setting up with a bowl in bed, or supervision when bathing, or help with one item of clothing, or help to shave).
3 Cannot manage independently in more than one or all aspects of personal hygiene (e.g. cannot wash self, or cannot dress self, or needs lifting into bath). May be very depressed.
4 Cannot manage any aspect of washing or dressing (e.g. is paralysed, unconscious, very confused, or a baby).

Wound care
1 No wound <u>or</u> can self–care.
2 Has a clean surgical wound causing minimal discomfort and inconvenience.
3 Has a wound which causes pain or inter–feres moderately with other activities of living (e.g. dressing, washing, mobilis–ing, sleeping, working and playing).

4 Has an extensive wound, which may cause severe pain or strongly influence ALs as above, plus breathing, communicating, sexuality, eating and drinking, or eliminating.

Skin care
1 Has clean intact skin or can manage skin care independently.
2 Is vulnerable to skin damage or cannot apply topical treatments to lesions.
3 Has a pressure sore which requires nursing intervention but nutritional state is good and can understand rationale for care.
4 Has a pressure sore as above but physical and/or mental state is poor.

CONTROLLING BODY TEMPERATURE

1 Temperature is within the normal range. Can cope with changes in environmental temperature.
2 Has mild pyrexia but is mentally alert and orientated.
3 Cannot physically/intellectually cope with changes in environmental temperature (e.g. is at either extreme of age).
4 Has hyperpyrexia or hypothermia or is unconscious.

Note The ALs of personal cleansing and dressing and controlling body temperature each have only four criteria for assessment.

Maintaining a safe environment

Annie said she coped perfectly well usually, and was annoyed about falling. She did her own housework, cooking and shopping with no problems. A potential problem in this activity after discharge was identified.

121

Communication

Annie was alert and orientated; she understood what had happened and expressed herself coherently. She did not seem particularly anxious, but regarded it as a nuisance which might interfere with her usual activities for some time. She was slightly deaf but wore no hearing aid; she wore bifocal spectacles.

Breathing

There was no history of respiratory problems, she had never smoked and seldom had colds. Apart from potential problems of the respiratory tract after anaesthetic or while on bed rest, no actual problems were identified.

Eating and drinking

Annie said she enjoyed her food, had a good appetite, never had indigestion and had never been overweight. She made no concessions to 'healthy' eating, and continued to eat what she liked. Her dislikes included 'new-fangled' foreign food. No problems were identified.

Eliminating

A vaginal repair ten years before had completely cured stress incontinence which Annie had suffered for several years previously. Her bowel pattern was regular, usually daily, and no actual problems were identified. Potential problems were related to difficulties of elimination while her mobility was reduced and she was being nursed in bed.

Personal cleansing and dressing

Annie said she took a bath at home independently with no problems. This might become more difficult for her after discharge and would need reassessing then. She appeared clean and well cared for. Due to her alert mental state, good physical condition and continence, the score on the Norton scale on admission was 15: this would need reassessing after operation. Annie had a full set of dentures. A potential problem of skin damage was identified.

Controlling body temperature

Temperature on admission was 36.4 °C. The clothes she had been wearing were appropriate for the time of year and no problems were identified.

Mobilising

This activity would be the focus of her nursing care. Usually fully mobile, she was now totally unable to walk, or to move about the bed freely due to discomfort and skin traction. After the operation her mobility would be limited for several days and she would need extensive rehabilitation. Pain and a change in usual mobilising were identified as actual problems.

Working and playing

Annie had not worked outside the home since her marriage fifty-six years ago. She received a state pension and a small pension from her husband's firm. She enjoyed gardening, cooking and reading, and belonged to a church fellowship group. She was on good terms with her neighbours. Her son usually visited her once a fortnight and took her to his home for Sunday lunch every month, when she saw her daughter-in-law. One grandson visited frequently but she hadn't seen the older one since his wedding and had never seen her great-grandchild. She seemed doubtful about help after discharge. She said her house was easy to manage, but had no downstairs lavatory and had steps between the bathroom and the bedrooms. Although a churchgoer she did not feel the need for communion or a chaplain while in hospital. Potential problems of coping after discharge were identified.

Expressing sexuality

Annie obviously cared for her appearance, and kept herself clean and fresh. No problems were identified.

Sleeping

Annie usually retired after the ten o'clock news on television and was up by 07.00. She woke during the night but never took sleeping tablets. No problems were identified.

Dying

When asked if she had any particular anxieties about the operation Annie said that if she got over it she hoped it would be completely successful, otherwise it would be better to die now. She had no fears about dying and would be ready when the time came. No problems were identified.

NURSING CARE

Routine pre- and post-operative care was explained to Annie and carried out as prescribed. Details are not described below for this care; routine post-operative care and care given to prevent complications are addressed fully in Chapter 4.

Annie went to theatre the morning after admission for insertion of a dynamic hip screw into the neck of the right femur. Her temperature on return to the ward was 35 °C but rose to 36 °C within four hours. Research by Closs *et al.* (1986) revealed that patients with a fractured femur lose more body heat in the peri-operative period than those undergoing abdominal surgery, especially if they are thin, so frequent recordings are recommended.

Annie's condition otherwise remained satisfactory. Post-operative analgesia was given as precribed. The emphasis below is on mobilising, communicating, eliminating, personal cleansing and dressing, and working and playing, which are described in the text and in graphs.

Eliminating; eating and drinking

These activities were considered together because it seemed difficult to separate them logically. Annie had not passed urine by 24 hours post-op. despite the usual encouragement so a urethral catheter was inserted and left on free drainage. This was explained to Annie. The long-term goal was for her to pass urine normally and for her urine to remain free from infection. Annie seemed mildly confused during this period and pulled the catheter out twice, so fluid balance was not recorded very accurately. Her intravenous infusion was continued until the fourth day as it was difficult to encourage her to drink although she ate a small diet well. Her son said she drank very little at home anyway. Annie was told her catheter and IVI would be removed when she could drink a little more; drinks were offered hourly and taken fairly well. The catheter was removed on the fifth day, after which she passed urine but was occasionally incontinent. Walsh and Ford (1989) cite research by Summerskill (1976) which indicated that because of long periods of nil by mouth, patients often become dehydrated in the 24 hours pre-op. which may cause mental confusion and electrolyte imbalance: in view of Annie's usual habits this may have been one cause of her confusion. By discharge on 27 February she was fully continent.

Personal cleansing and dressing

There were two problems in this activity: first, normally independent, Annie had moved towards the dependent pole for personal hygiene activities post-operatively; second, she was completely dependent on nursing intervention for care of her wound. The long-term goals were that she would regain her former level of independence in washing and dressing, and her wound would heal within twelve days with no signs of infection.

Nursing actions and evaluation   Annie was given a bed bath on the first day post-op. Subsequently she was encouraged to do as much as possible for herself in bed or in a bedside chair. She was told that if all went well she would have a bath after her sutures had been removed on day 12. Due to her mild confusion in the first few days, Annie needed help with washing. She bathed on day 12 using a bath board and scat, as planned, with minimal assistance; by discharge four days later, however, she still required some help for this activity.

The wound was stripped and steripads applied after 48 hours: research by Thomlinson (1987) shows that taking down the dressing earlier may introduce infection as skin will not have formed a protective barrier. Steripads were renewed as necessary. Wound drainage was recorded daily for 72 hours, after which the drain was removed. The suture line became inflamed and tender on day 5, with considerable exudate. Annie's temperature was 37.8 °C. Antibiotic therapy was commenced, based on a bacteriology report; the wound was cleaned daily and re-dressed with Debrisan absorbent pad. By day 12 the wound was cleaner, with less inflammation and exudate, so sutures were removed on the doctor's instructions leaving 5 cm (2 in.) at the proximal end of the suture line gaping.

Wound care and supervision when bathing were identified as continuing problems after discharge, and the community nurse was asked to dress Annie's wound.

Mobilising

Annie was unable to mobilise as usual due to pain and to the prescribed regime following this operation. This was the focal problem, and it influenced most other activities. One long-term goal was that Annie should be able to mobilise freely within twelve or fourteen days, which in her case would include managing at least one flight of stairs. The short-term goals set to meet this may be seen in her care plan. The other goal was that Annie would not develop complications of bed rest.

Nursing actions and evaluation   The nurse's role in preventive care is illustrated by the care given to prevent complication of bed rest. Annie's skin remained intact and no signs of chest infection or deep vein thrombosis developed. After being seen by doctors on her second post-op. day to establish stable fixation (there always being a potential problem of instability of the hip fixation), she was helped by a nurse and physiotherapist to stand; from then on she was encouraged to walk increasing distances each day, first with two helpers, then with one person, and ultimately with a frame or sticks for support.

Annie had very little confidence and was reluctant to walk without a nurse, but by her fourteenth day she was managing to get around the ward satisfactorily with minimal discomfort, using her frame. She was less confident on stairs, which caused anxiety. This was identified as a continuing problem on discharge. Her son said that normally she was energetic and independent and thought she was making slow progress.

Working and playing

Annie's lifestyle would need modification after discharge, and anxiety about this was the main problem. This activity provided the focus for discharge planning. Her son and daughter-in-law did not offer any help on discharge, but the son would continue his usual visits. A social worker visited Annie but her son declined to see her, feeling that relevant information could be communicated via his mother or the ward sister. A home visit with the social worker and occupational therapist was arranged with Annie and she managed walking and stairs better at home, although still not at her previous level of independence and safety. As a temporary measure her son agreed to move a bed downstairs for her and to borrow a commode, so that all activities could be carried out on one level. He also arranged for a telephone by her bed and agreed to look into the possibility of bath rails. A neighbour offered to call daily to empty the commode; a home help was organised for once a week; and meals-on-wheels were to be provided three days a week. Annie was not happy about this but was persuaded to accept this arrangement. She would try to cook for herself on the other days.

DISCHARGE

Annie was discharged home on the afternoon of her sixteenth day, a Monday, with a bath seat, a bath board and a raised lavatory seat for when she was able to get upstairs. The community nurse was asked to dress the wound; the district physiotherapist arranged to continue helping Annie to practise stairs, and a social services care attendant was arranged to help with a weekly bath. Annie's understanding of all the follow-up arrangements and her medication was checked. She would be seen as an out-patient in six weeks' time, and transport was arranged for this.

Because she was still not fully independently mobilising, she had not returned to the independent pole of this continuum for eating and drinking, eliminating, personal cleansing and dressing or working and playing.

Nursing care at home

The community nurse visited Annie the day after discharge. Her assessment was based on the discharge note and on observation and information from Annie. See Figure 7.5 (page 144) for her assessment of ALs.

Maintaining a safe environment

Annie was not safe to use the stairs alone or to bathe. There was a potential problem of further accidents because of unsteadiness. Advice and observation were required, but no accidents apart from a slight slip in the bath were reported.

Communication

Annie seemed depressed. This was not identified as a problem at the first visit and did not persist.

Eating and drinking

Annie was still not happy about meals-on-wheels. She had made her own breakfast but said her appetite had not returned. (She had eaten well in hospital.) This was identified as a potential problem which might need close observation. In fact Annie cancelled meals-on-wheels after only two weeks and managed well. Her neighbour and grandson helped with shopping.

Eliminating

Annie was not happy about the commode but her neighbour had been very helpful. Although this was not identified as a problem at once, on her visit the care attendant noticed that Annie seemed to have some dribbling urinary incontinence. She asked about her bowels and there was also some faecal leaking, although she had not had a proper bowel action since discharge. This was reported to the district nurse and faecal impaction identified, and cleared with two disposable enemata.

Personal cleansing and dressing

Annie had washed at the kitchen sink but was not happy about this either. She asked when she could have help with bathing and the district nurse explained her role and that of the care attendant who would time her first visit with that of the physiotherapist, to learn how Annie managed stairs. Thereafter the care attendant called weekly to help her upstairs and with the bath. Annie made quick progress with stairs and her bed was moved upstairs again two weeks after discharge. She remained nervous about bathing, as she had slipped the first time she tried. She then arranged to take a bath when someone was in the house, in case she fell.

The proximal end of her wound was granulating and the remaining suture line was clean and intact. Annie had occasional pain in the wound. The goal for the wound was that it would continue to granulate and heal without further infection within two weeks. The wound was dressed daily for two days, then every other day with Debrisan for one week, after which there was very little exudate and it looked clean with increased granulation. After this it was re-dressed with a simple dressing until completely dry and healed, which took another ten days. By this time Annie was feeling much stronger and dressed it herself. The nurse made two further weekly visits, stopping her calls at the end of March.

Mobilising

Annie was frustrated by her slowness but realistic about her abilities and future potential. The problem of her not having returned to full independence in mobilising was identified, and intervention would consist of observation only. A return to independence in mobilising was reflected in progress in other activities.

Controlling body temperature

February was a cold month but the house had gas central heating which had been set by her son to automatic. It was not on at night, but she preferred it that way. In the event of a fall at night a cold bedroom might be a threat to her well-being: this was explained to her and identified as a potential problem. Intervention consisted of advice and observation only.

Working and playing

Annie seemed embarrassed to talk about her son and his lack of help and made many excuses. The subject was not pursued. During the visit, Annie's younger grandson, Paul, called. He and his girlfriend worked close by and planned to call in at least once a day to see her, and perhaps to shop, to change her library books, or to give her a run out in the car. Annie was visibly cheered by this, and no problems were identified for the present.

No other activities of living were assessed.

Annie attended for her follow-up appointment six weeks after discharge and was discharged. One week later her neighbour noticed that Annie's bedroom curtains were still pulled late morning: she went in and found Annie unconscious on the bedroom floor. Annie was re-admitted at 11.00 via A&E to the elderly care ward at the same hospital, following a cerebral vascular accident. Between the ages of sixty and ninety thrombosis is the most common cause, often occurring during sleep or after rising due to brain ischaemia caused by recumbency (Long and Phipps 1985).

Annie was accompanied by her grandson, who had been contacted by the neighbour. Assessment was based on observation, the medical notes, and information from the grandson (Figure 7.6, page 145). Primary nursing is carried out on this twenty-bed Nightingale-type ward and assessment was carried out by the nurse allocated to Annie, who introduced herself as Alison and briefly explained about primary nursing. Paul was pleased to be included in planning Annie's care. All care was explained to him. Breathing and tempera-ture were described as priorities. The care plan is shown in Figure 7.7 (pages 146–53).

Breathing

Annie was breathing independently but she was dependent on others for maintenance of a clear airway. Potential problems of an obstruc-ted airway and chest infection were identified. She was nursed in a semi-prone position and excess secretions were cleared by suction; the apparatus and airway were kept by her bed all the time. Her breathing remained shallow, with a respiration rate between 14 and 18 per minute. Oxygen was administered as prescribed.

Controlling body temperature

Annie's rectal temperature was 32.4 °C on admission. (She was thought to have been on the floor since the early hours of the morning.) Hypothermia is said to exist when the body temperature is below 35 °C (Roberts 1989). The goal was for the temperature to increase by 0.5 °C per hour until 36 °C was reached in about six hours. Pulse, blood pressure and rectal temperature were recorded half-hourly until the temperature reached 34 °C; and hourly until it had been stable at 36.2 °C for two observations, after which the space blanket was removed.

Maintaining a safe environment

Annie was unconscious and therefore fully dependent on others to maintain her safety. Nursing care consisted of frequent observation and the use of padded cotsides on the bed at all times.

Communication

Annie was totally unable to communicate. Although she remained unconscious her family were encouraged to touch her and talk to her as though she could hear them, because it is always possible that hearing persists during unconsciousness. Her son felt this was unnecessary and restricted his daily visit to a quick glance and a word with the nurse in charge. Paul visited frequently, talking to her freely. He felt sure she understood him.

Eating and drinking

Annie had no swallow reflex so an actual problem of needing feeding by artificial routes was identified. A goal for fluid intake (100 ml per hour) was established and a nasogastric tube had been passed in A&E. Nursing care involved care of the tube, maintaining the fluid regime as prescribed by medical staff, and recording the fluid balance. Annie remained unconscious and the nasogastric tube remained *in situ* throughout the four days with no obvious discomfort. There is a danger of hypovolaemic shock occurring with vasodilation in hypothermia, so intravenous fluids were not introduced (Long and Phipps 1985).

Eliminating

An actual problem of urinary incontinence was identified and potential problems of constipation or faecal incontinence were considered. The goal was for Annie to remain clean, dry and comfortable. A urethral catheter was inserted and left on free drainage using a closed system. The catheter and vulval area were washed regularly and output was recorded. Output decreased over the four days. Rectal examination revealed small hard faeces and two glycerine suppositories were given with effect. No further bowel action was recorded.

Mobilising

Annie was totally dependent on nurses for position changes. Potential problems of complications of bed rest, and limb contractures were identified; both would require preventive nursing. The score on the Norton scale was 7, indicating a high risk for pressure-sore development (Norton *et al.* 1962). Annie was nursed on an alternating pressure mattress, her pressure areas observed and her position changed from side to side two-hourly. A chart adapted from Lowthian's turning clock was used to record turn times (Lowthian 1979). Annie's limbs were supported in a position of rest at each turn to avoid contractures. The skin over the malleoli looked red at each turn so sheepskin bootees were used from the second day.

Personal cleansing and dressing

Annie required total nursing care for this activity and the long-term goal was for her to look clean and preserve her dignity, although she was unconscious. All hygiene activities were carried out when necessary, taking care not to disturb her unnecessarily. Her own toiletries were used, and she wore her own nightdresses. Her mouth was kept clean and moist and Vaseline was applied to her lips. Her eyes became 'sticky' frequently and were swabbed with normal saline as necessary.

Sleeping

In the model, the level of consciousness is included in this AL, although in Annie's care plan it is recorded in the AL of maintaining a safe environment. Neurological observations were carried out with other observations, first half-hourly and then hourly for the first 48 hours, using the Glasgow coma scale. Annie's level of consciousness varied little in the next four days. During the first three days she sometimes opened her eyes and made slight movements in response to painful stimuli, but she made no verbal response.

Dying

Paul asked if Annie would die. Alison, the nurse, spoke to him about this possibility. He was obviously very fond of his grandmother and said he had never experienced anyone dying. Anxiety and sadness of the family was identified as an actual problem.

As there had been no observable change in her condition none of her family was with her when she died at 22.45 on 18 April. Paul was informed at once, as requested, but did not want to see her; her son was told the following morning. He had not expected her to recover and seemed philosophical about her death, but was concerned with practical details (which may have been his way of coping with his feelings). Paul visited the ward with chocolates one week later and talked about his grandmother. Alison told him when she would be on duty and invited him to pop in if he wanted to talk at any time, but he did not do so.

SUMMARY

Annie's care was carried out in three different areas using this model, which illustrates how the roles of the nurse change to meet the changing needs of the patient. The dependent and interdependent roles are demonstrated by liaison with medical staff, social workers, physiotherapists, the care attendant and the family. The AL component is in evidence in care given to prevent complications of surgery, bed rest, and immobility; also by encouraging Annie to eat and drink. The psychosocial, physical and developmental influences on the ALs were recognised in assessing and discharge planning, and principles of holism are emphasised by acknowledging the needs of the family. Annie's changing status on the dependence–independence continuum was recorded using a ward-devised scale to give more accurate assessment and evaluation for each AL.

EXERCISES AND ACTIVITIES

Exercise 1

Aim   To compare pressure-sore risk, using two different scales.

Method   Individual work, on ward; recording results.

Resources   Five patients; Waterlow risk card and Norton scale; paper or charts.

Suggested time   If tools are available, allow two weeks to collect data, tabulate results and write a rationale.

1 Select five patients in your care. Assess their pressure-sore risk using each scale. Tabulate and interpret your results. Compare the levels of risk indicated by each score with that indicated by your own clinical observation.

2 Write a report on your findings.

  • Which tool is simpler to use?
  • Which tool did you think was more accurate?
  • Give a rationale for your choice.

Exercise 2

Aim   To apply the principle of the dependence–independence continuum to assessing patient dependence.

Method   Daily assessments; timing nurse interventions; individual and group work.

Resources   Guideline (Figure 7.1); one patient.

133

Suggested time   2 weeks for assessing and timing; 1 hour to create a recording form in the group.

1 In groups of three or four:

- List all the interventions required to enable the patient to carry out each AL as described in the guideline (Figure 7.1).
- Create a form on which to record times for each intervention listed.

2 Individually:

- Using the guidelines, for one week record the daily dependencies of a patient of your choice in the eight ALs represented in the guide: minimum possible score = 10 (most independent); maximum possible score = 46 (most dependent).

  Dependency categories may be obtained as follows:

10	Category 1
11–22	Category 2
23–34	Category 3
25–46	Category 4

- If you are already measuring patient dependency at your hospital, compare the patient's category with that arrived at with the tool already in use. If not, compare the category you have obtained for your patient with your own observational assessment of his/her dependency needs.
- Over a period of one shift record the time taken to carry out each intervention. Add up the totals.

3 In the same group of three or four:

- Compare timings. Do they make sense? Discussion could include: aspects of direct nursing care not covered by the guideline; aspects of indirect nursing care not considered; other ways of assessing dependence.

Exercise 3

Aim   To apply knowledge of developmental aspects of the model to care planning.

Method   Individual work.

Resources   Care planning documents.

Suggested time   1 hour 30 minutes.

134

1 Select a patient in a particular age group for whom to assess, plan and evaluate care using this model.

2 List the ALs which are particularly influenced by the position on the life span, and those which would remain the same for any age group.

3 Discuss how this has influenced care planning.

Figure 7.2

PATIENT ASSESSMENT FORM	Biographical and health

Date of admission 11th February
Date of assessment 11th February   Signature J. Bone

Patient
Surname COLEMAN   Forename(s) ANNIE ROSE
~~Male~~   Age 78   Prefers to be
Female   DOB 10/07/12   addressed as Annie

Usual address 27 Goldsmith Terrace, Charbridge

Type of accommodation Terraced house

Others at this residence None

Next of kin
Name Donald Coleman   Relationship Son
Address 5 Oak Crescent,
Glebelands Park, Charbridge Telephone number Charbridge 567892

Significant others Paul Coleman (grandson)

Occupation Housewife

Religious beliefs Churchgoer: C of E.
and practices

Recent significant Death of husband 5 years ago.
life crises

Patient's perception Good up till now.
of current health

Family's perception Have noticed no change.
of current health

Medical information Childhood illnesses; vaginal repair 10
years ago; 1 normal pregnancy. ? Mild CVA 2 years ago.
Taking Aprinox 2.5mg for hypertension. Suspects she is
allergic to tinned fish.

GP
Name Dr Wood
Address City Health Centre
          Telephone number Charbridge 654321

Consultant Mr Oak

Discharge plans Will need contact with community nurse.
May require home help and meals on wheels. Will
need bath and lavatory aids.

136

Figure 7.3

PATIENT ASSESSMENT FORM		Assessment of ALs	
Name Annie Coleman		Date of birth 10/07/12	
Stage of care Admission		Date of assessment 11/02	
		Signature J. Bone	
Activity of living	**Usual routine**	**Problems** A : Actual P : Potential	
Maintaining a safe environment	Independent	Complications of surgery/bed rest (P). Unable to walk freely due to # neck of rt. femur.	
Communicating	No speech or hearing problems. Wears bifocal glasses.	Mild anxiety about operation and its effects (P).	
Breathing	No respiratory problems Non-smoker.	Breathing problems after operation (P).	
Eating and drinking	Good appetite. Sherry before dinner.	No problems.	
Eliminating	Regular bowel pattern. No urinary problems.	Difficulties in eliminating due to limited mobility (P)	
Personal cleansing and dressing	Fully independent.	Wound infection, skin damage post-op. Difficulty due to limited mobility (P). Norton scale = 15.	
Controlling body temperature	Fully independent.		
Mobilising	Fully independent.	Limited mobility pre- and post-op. (A).	
Working and playing	Housewife. Church fellowship. Outings with son.	Anxiety about being unable to cope as usual (A).	
Expressing sexuality	Clean appearance. Post-menopausal.	No problems.	
Sleeping	Usually about 8 hrs per night. Wakes a lot.	No problems.	
Dying	Discusses possibility openly.	No problems.	

Figure 7.4

NURSING CARE PLAN related to ALs	
Name ANNIE COLEMAN	**Date of birth** 10/07/12
Stage of care	**Date** 12th Feb. *Signature* J. Bone

AL EATING AND DRINKING	DR 3

Problem(s) unable to eat and drink as usual after operation (A)
Dehydration (P).

Long-term goal(s) To return by discharge to previous independence in eating and drinking.

Goal	Actions	Evaluation
24 hr fluid intake to be 2 litres. IVI to run as prescribed. Site to be comfortable with no soreness.	Observe IVI and site with other obs. Record fluid balance.	12/02. 20.00. IVI as prescribed. Taking sips of water. J.B.
To tolerate free oral fluids and light diet by 14th. Mouth to feel moist and clean.	Offer sips of water when awake, increase amounts as tolerated. Offer mouthwashes PRN.	13/02. Reluctant to drink, sips only taken. J.B.
	14/02 Explain that IVI can come down when she is drinking more. Offer 100 ml water/fruit juice hourly, as well as tea. K.C	14/02 No change: total oral intake only 300 ml. DR=4. Small diet taken. K.C.
		15/02 Drinking well, IVI discont. 15.00. DR=2. K.C.

138

Figure 7.4 (continued)

NURSING CARE PLAN	related to ALs	
Name ANNIE COLEMAN	Date of birth 10/07/12	
Stage of care	Date 13th Feb. Signature S. Bone	

AL ELIMINATING DR 4

Problem(s) Has not passed urine post-op. (A)
Constipation (P)
Long-term goal(s) To return by discharge to normal patterns of elimination.

Goal	Actions	Evaluation
To pass at least 1500 ml urine in 24 hrs. Catheter to drain freely, urine to remain free from infection.	Insert catheter size 12, leave on free drainage. Explain reasons, check understanding. Observe urine, record output.	14/02 Annie pulled catheter out x 2 Reinserted, draining well. K.C.
17/02 To pass urine within 6 hrs of catheter removal.	16/02 For a trial run without catheter from 17/02. J.B.	17/02 Has PU. Fluid balance recorded, output satisfactory. Incontinent urine x 2. Still confused: DR = 3. J.B.
18/02 To ask for bedpan/commode each time she wants to PU.	Make sure Annie has her call bell at hand. Offer bedpan 3 hrly. REVIEW 20/02	20/02 Continent today. Bowels open. 21/02 Incont urine x1 J.B.
	26/02 Check with occupational therapist re high loo seat for home. J.B.	26/02 Continent since 21st. Manages with high loo seat. DR = 2. J.B.

139

Figure 7.4 (continued)

NURSING CARE PLAN related to ALs	
Name ANNIE COLEMAN	**Date of birth** 10/07/12
Stage of care	**Date** 13th Feb.
	Signature J Bone

AL PERSONAL CLEANSING AND DRESSING   **DR** 3

Problem(s) 1. Unable to wash and dress herself for short time after operation.

Long-term goal(s) To return to previous level of independence by discharge or day 14.

Goal	Actions	Evaluation
Annie will look and feel fresh and clean at all times and start to wash herself, with help, from day 2.	Give bed bath on day 1. Encourage Annie to wash herself as much as possible from day 2. REVIEW daily. Help with bath in bathroom after suture removal: ? day 12	14/02 Confused, could not wash herself. K.C. 15/02 Emptied her juice in washing water and washed locker with flannel. K.C. 17/02 Less confused, washed thoroughly. J.B.
	24/02 Check bath board and seat supplied for discharge. K.C.	24/02 Managed bath with minimal help. Quite pleased with herself. DR = 2. K.C.

Figure 7.4 (continued)

NURSING CARE PLAN	related to ALs	
Name ANNIE COLEMAN		Date of birth 10/07/12
Stage of care		Date 12th Feb.
		Signature S. Bone

AL PERSONAL CLEANSING AND DRESSING   DR 3

Problem(s) 2. Potential wound infection

Long-term goal(s) Wound to heal without infection by day 12.

Goal	Actions	Evaluation
Suture line to remain intact with no redness, exudate or increased tenderness. REVIEW daily.	Dressing to remain in situ for 48 hrs. 14/02 Strip wound, clean with normal saline, apply steripads. Renew if uncomfortable or wet or if Annie is pyrexial. Empty drainage and read amount daily. K-C 17/02 Dress with Debrisan absorbent pad. Renew when soaked with exudate. SB 22/02 Take wound swab when antibiotic course completed. LD 24/02 Refer to community nurse for continued care. K-C	13/02 Dressing comfortable, drainage recorded. J.S 14/02 Wound looks clean. Drainage 150 ml. K-C 15/02 Drainage 75 ml. Drain removed on Dr's instructions. K-C 16/02 Drain site oozing. Redressed. S.B. 17/02 Suture line red and tender. Purulent exudate proximal end. Temp 37.8°C. Wound swab taken. J.B 18/02 Wound inflamed, tender. Less exudate. Antibiotics started. J.S 20/02 Less inflamed. Proximal sutures still 'sticky'. S.B. 22/02 Alternate sutures removed on Dr's instructions. Wound swab taken. LD 24/02 Proximal end gaping slightly. All sutures removed, re-dressed. DR=3. K-C

141

Figure 7.4 (continued)

NURSING CARE PLAN	related to ALs	
Name ANNIE COLEMAN		**Date of birth** 10/07/12
Stage of care		**Date** 13th Feb
		Signature J. Bone
AL MOBILISING		**DR** 5

Problem(s) Unable to mobilise freely due to pain and prescribed post-operative regime.

Long-term goal(s) Annie will be able to walk around ward freely and manage one flight of stairs by 25th Feb.

Goal	Actions	Evaluation
To remain free from skin damage. DVT and chest infection The hip joint to remain stable with no increase of pain on movement.	Observe pressure areas and help Annie to change position 2 hrly while in bed. Observe calves for redness or tenderness daily. Encourage exercises taught by physios.	20/02 No complications of bed rest have developed. Continue to observe. J.B.
To be able to transfer from bed to chair unaided by 16/02.	16/02 Help Annie out of bed with physio. after seen by Drs. J.B.	16/02. Annie still mildly confused did not help herself much. J.B.
To be able to walk around bed area un-aided with frame by 18/02.	17/02 2 nurses to help to walk in bed area only. Increase distance daily. J.B.	18/02 Not at all confident. Reluctant to walk alone. DR = 3 J.B
To walk with frame to lavatory unaided by 20/02.	Arrange home visit with social worker for 25/02. J.B.	20/02. Still lacks confidence. Says she will manage once she gets home. J.B.
To walk freely with frame and manage stairs by 24/02.		24/02 Walked to bathroom with frame. Managed well. K.C.
		25/02 Did well on home visit but not safe on stairs. DR = 2. J.B

142

Figure 7.4 (continued)

NURSING CARE PLAN related to ALs	
Name ANNIE COLEMAN	**Date of birth** 10/07/12
Stage of care	**Date** 20th Feb.
	Signature S. Bone

AL WORKING AND PLAYING   **DR**

Problem(s) Needs to modify lifestyle after discharge until she can manage all ALs safely.

Long-term goal(s) Annie will manage safely at home (to be evaluated by community staff).

Goal	Actions	Evaluation
To demonstrate ability to carry out ALs safely and independently.	Refer to physio's report and care plans above. Check bath seat, board. (oo seat and TTOs have been supplied. (Son is getting commode.)	Annie cannot manage stairs or bath safely. District physio to visit. Social worker organised meals-on-wheels, home help, care attendant for bath. Referred to community nurse for wound care. S.B.
Annie and family to demonstrate understanding and to be able to discuss arrangements confidently.	Keep informed about all follow-up arrangements. Explain medications. Ask Annie to paraphrase all information. Allow time for questions.	Annie and son aware of arrangements. Annie not happy about commode or meals-on-wheels but was persuaded to agree. S.B.

143

Figure 7.5

PATIENT ASSESSMENT FORM	Assessment of ALs
Community nurse	

Name ANNIE COLEMAN	Date of birth 10/07/12
Stage of care	Date of assessment 28/02
	Signature P. Chan

Activity of living	Usual routine	Problems A : Actual P : Potential
Maintaining a safe environment	Still not totally confident on stairs since operation.	Falls (P)
Communicating	Able to communicate well. Slightly deaf.	Depression (P)
Breathing		
Eating and drinking	Has meals-on-wheels 3x a week. Says she has no appetite.	Lack of nutrients for wound-healing (P)
Eliminating	Uses commode in downstairs bedroom. Needs help to empty commode.	Dislikes using commode (P)
Personal cleansing and dressing	Wound not healed, slight pain. Unable to bathe independently.	Wound infection (P); lack of independence (A)
Controlling body temperature	Has central heating, but not at night	Hypothermia (P)
Mobilising	Unable to move freely due to nature of operation and lack of confidence. Norton scale 16	Frustration at limitations and dependence on others (A)
Working and playing	Grandson will visit, shop and take her out. Neighbour visits daily.	No problems
Expressing sexuality		
Sleeping		
Dying		

144

Figure 7.6

PATIENT ASSESSMENT FORM	Assessment of ALs	
Name ANNIE COLEMAN	**Date of birth** 10 107 /12	
Stage of care	**Date of assessment** 14th April	
	Signature A. Douglas	
Activities of living	**Problems**	
	Actual	**Potential**
Maintaining a safe environment	Unconscious. Fully dependent.	Not able to maintain safety in any AL.
Communicating	No verbal communication Very occasional motor response.	May have pain.
Breathing	Stertorous respiration Unable to keep own airway clear.	Respiratory tract infection.
Eating and drinking	Absent swallow reflex.	Dehyaration.
Eliminating	Incontinence of urine. No urinary problems	Constipation and/or faecal incontinence.
Personal cleansing and dressing	Fully dependent. Sticky eyes.	Skin damage. Dry mouth.
Controlling body temperature	Hypothermia	Circulatory collapse due to sudden rise in temp.
Mobilising	Fully dependent. Norton scale = 7.	Limb contractures. Deep vein thrombosis.
Working and playing		
Expressing sexuality		
Sleeping	Glasgow Coma scale = 6. Open eyes, moves arm in response to pain only occasionally.	
Dying	Grandson is anxious about her dying.	

145

Figure 7.7

NURSING CARE PLAN related to ALs	
Name ANNIE COLEMAN	**Date of birth** 10/07/12
Stage of care	**Date** 14th April **Signature** A Douglas

AL   BREATHING   **DR**

Problem(s) Unable to maintain own airway (A). Obstructed airway, chest infection (P).
Long-term goal(s) Airway to remain clear. No chest infection.

Goal	Actions	Evaluation
No cyanosis, respiratory distress or increased restlessness.	Nurse in semi-prone position. Ensure airway and suction by bed. Observe/record resps half-hrly. Review BD. Administer oxygen as instructed PRN. 17/04 Oxygen given as instructed. _A D_	14/04 Shallow resps, 14-18 per min. Suction used PRN. No cyanosis, a little restless. _A D_ 15/04 a.m. No change. _A D_ 18.00 Bubbly respirations, frequent suction needed. No cyanosis. _A D_ 16/04 a.m. No change in nature or rate of resps BE 19.00 - as above BE 17/04 11.00 As above. Cyanosed extremities. _A D_ 19.00 Cheyne Stokes respirations observed BE 18/04 Cheyne Stokes continues _H D_ 22.45 Breathing ceased. F.C.

Figure 7.7 (continued)

NURSING CARE PLAN   related to ALs

Name ANNIE COLEMAN	Date of birth 10/07/12
Stage of care	Date 14th April
	Signature A. Douglas

AL MAINTAINING A SAFE ENVIRONMENT   **DR**

Problem(s) Unconscious. Unable to maintain own safety. Score on Glasgow coma scale = 6.

Long-term goal(s) To return to consciousness.

Goal	Actions	Evaluation
Alterations in level of consciousness to be recognised promptly.	Neuro obs. using Glasgow coma scale half-hrly. Review BD.	14/04 18.00 No change since admission. A.D
Annie to remain free from injury while unconscious.	Keep padded cotsides in situ whenever no one is with her.	15/04 06.00 Score 6. See chart A.D
		19.00 As above. Seems quite peaceful. Grandson with her. A.D
	16/04 Continue to obs. hourly. Review chart. BE	16/04 am. No change BE
		17/04 ?Some verbal response (reported by grandson). Not clear; not repeated. A.D
		18/04 Score 4. No change all day. A.D

147

Figure 7.7 (continued)

NURSING CARE PLAN related to ALs	
Name ANNIE COLEMAN	**Date of birth** 10/07/12
Stage of care	**Date** 14th April **Signature** A. Douglas

AL COMMUNICATING   **DR**

Problem(s) Unconscious. Unable to make needs known.

Long-term goal(s) To have all her needs met while unconscious.

Goal	Actions	Evaluation
Any signs of pain, discomfort or distress to be identified promptly.	Talk to Annie as though conscious. Make use of touch. Observe closely for any response. Encourage family to talk to her, explain that she might be able to hear.	15/04 Annie seems peaceful, no response observed. Visited by son and grandson. Grandson thinks she understands him. A.D

148

Figure 7.7 (continued)

NURSING CARE PLAN	related to ALs
Name ANNIE COLEMAN	**Date of birth** 10/07/12
Stage of care	**Date** 14th April
	Signature A. Douglas
AL EATING AND DRINKING	**DR**

Problem(s) Absent swallow reflex (A). Fluid overload, hypovolaemic shock (P).

Long-term goal(s) Nutrition and fluid balance to be maintained while unconscious.

Goal	Actions	Evaluation
Fluid balance to be maintained.	Adjust intake daily according to 24 hr output. 75ml per hour. Record intake and output. Aspirate NG tube 2 hrly. Nasogastric tube to remain in situ. Give feeds as regime. Test reaction of aspirate. Ensure tube is securely attached to face.	15/04 NG tube in situ. Aspirated before feeds. feeds as prescribed. Annie seems unaware of tube. A.D. 16/04 NG regime continued BE 17/04 Intake modified due to low urine output. A.D.

149

Figure 7.7 (continued)

NURSING CARE PLAN related to ALs	
Name ANNIE COLEMAN	**Date of birth** 10/07/12
Stage of care	**Date** 14th April *Signature* A Douglas

AL ELIMINATING   **DR**

Problem(s) Incontinent of urine (A). Incontinent of faeces/constipation (P)

Long-term goal(s) Annie will remain clean, dry and comfortable.

Goal	Actions	Evaluation
Catheter to drain freely, urine to remain infection-free.	Wash and dry perineum and round catheter PRN, at least BD. Empty drainage bag per shift, record intake and output.	15/04 24 hr urine output low (750 ml). Catheter draining well. Small hard faeces felt PR. Good result from supps A.D.
Lower rectum to be empty on rectal examination.	15/04 Give 2 glycerine suppositories stat. A.D	17/04 24 hr output decreased. A.D 18/04 Output very low (330 ml). Urine concentrated. A.D

150

Figure 7.7 (continued)

NURSING CARE PLAN related to ALs	
Name ANNIE COLEMAN	Date of birth 16/07/12
Stage of care	Date 14th April Signature A. Douglas

AL MOBILISING/PERSONAL CLEANSING AND DRESSING   **DR**

Problem(s) Norton scale score = 7. Unable to change position or carry out any personal hygiene activities (A). Limb contractures; skin damage (D).

Long-term goal(s) Annie will be comfortable and clean, and her dignity, preserved.

Goal	Actions	Evaluation
Skin to remain intact and not discoloured	Turn Annie 2 hrly. Record turns on clock chart. Nurse on alternating pressure bed.	15/04 Ankles looking red after 2 hours. Sheepskin bootees applied. A.D.
Limbs to remain flexible.	Arrange limbs in position of rest at each turn.	17/04 Pressure areas intact. Limbs flexible. A.D.
Annie to look fresh and clean.	Carry out all hygiene activities as needed with minimum disturbance. Use own talcum and toilet water.	18/04 Skin on sacrum looks red. Continue 2 hourly turns. A.D.

Figure 7.7 (continued)

NURSING CARE PLAN	related to ALs

Name ANNIE COLEMAN   **Date of birth** 10/07/12

Stage of care   **Date** 15th April
    Signature A. Douglas

AL CONTROLLING BODY TEMPERATURE   **DR**

Problem(s) Hypothermia (rectal temp. 32.4°C) due to lying unconscious on floor of unheated bedroom for several hours.

Long-term goal(s) Temperature to return to within normal range.

Goal	Actions	Evaluation
Temperature to rise by 0.5°C per hour until 36°C. BP to remain above 100/60 mm Hg. Pulse rate to remain 60-90 bpm. Review PRN at least 2 hrly at first	Wrap in space blanket. Record rectal temp half-hrly for 4 hours or until increasing regularly. Record BP and pulse rate with temperature	13.00 Rectal temp. 32.8°C, BP 106/60 mm Hg. Pulse 64 bpm. *A.D.*
		15.00 Rectal temp 33.6°C BP 110/65. Pulse 66. Continue TPR and BP half-hrly. *A.D.*
		18.00 Temp. 34°C. Continue hrly obs. BP/pulse stable *A.D.*
		22.00 Temp 35.8°C Continue hrly obs. *A.D.*
		16/04 06.00 Temp. 36.2°C since 12mn. Obs. reduced to 2hrly. *BE*
		18.00 Temp 36.6°C Continue obs. 4 hrly. *BE*
		17/04 No change in condition *A.D.*
		18/04 17.00 BP 90/55. Pulse 48 Drs informed. *A.D.*

152

Figure 7.7 (continued)

NURSING CARE PLAN	related to ALs

Name ANNIE COLEMAN	**Date of birth** 10/07/12
Stage of care	**Date** 15th April **Signature** A. Douglas

AL DYING		**DR**

Problem(s) Annie's family are anxious about her possible death (A).
Paul has no experence of death in the family.

Long-term goal(s)

Goal	Actions	Evaluation
Family to be able to express their feelings about Annie dying, and to be kept informed.	Allow time to talk to son and Paul. Provide privacy. Assess any special needs. Answer questions as honestly as possible.	Paul very sad that his grandmother might die and wants to be told at any time. A.D. 18/04 22.45 annie died peacefully. No family present, but notified as requested. F.C.

Figure 7.8 *A comparison of dependence–independence at three stages of care*

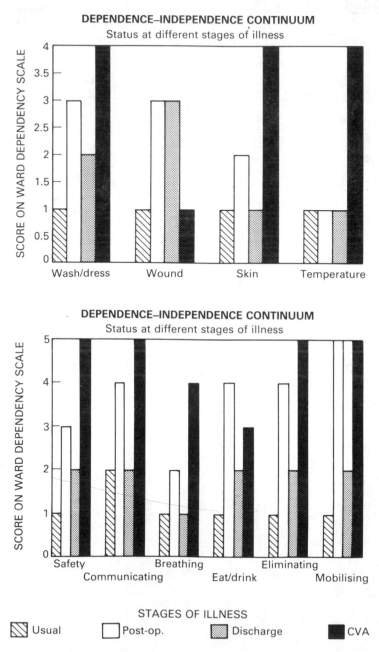

CHAPTER EIGHT

Care study: a young person with diabetes

Insulin-dependent diabetes mellitus, in which there is an absolute deficit of insulin, usually starts in younger people, who then need treatment for the rest of their lives. This chapter describes the care of a 19-year-old university student, Jody, over a period of five days during which she started to learn to manage her own care. She was nursed in a four-bedded bay on an acute medical ward; her primary nurse, John, was a diabetic himself so was particularly interested in the management of care related to diabetes.

MS JODY COLCROSS

Jody had visited her doctor, complaining of excessive thirst, weight loss of about a stone (6 kg) in four weeks, a need to pass urine more frequently, and increasing tiredness. A friend had suggested that she could be suffering from diabetes and this was confirmed after fasting blood-glucose tests. As she lived in a hall of residence at the university she was admitted to hospital while her insulin dosage was stabilised. Her nursing care would use teaching, counselling, and facilitating skills to help her learn how to test her blood and urine, to plan her diet, to administer her insulin, and to modify her usual activities of living to incorporate these new skills.

Wilson Barnett (1988) argues that the terms 'information-giving', 'teaching' and 'counselling' are used carelessly in nursing, which may lead to inadequate practice. She maintains that all patients need information about their illness; all patients with chronic or continuing illness need teaching to master new skills or modify present lifestyles; and some patients require further emotional support, or counselling, to cope. The emphasis in this chapter is on the factors that influenced the way Jody usually performed the ALs, and the

155

information, teaching and counselling planned to help her incorporate new ways of coping into her usual routine for living.

ADMISSION

Biographical details are given in Figure 8.1 (page 164). A full assessment of activities of living was carried out as soon as possible, and is described below and recorded in Figure 8.2 (page 165). As Jody had until now been a healthy girl of normal physiological and psychosocial development she was at the independent pole of the continuum for all ALs: it was the individual way in which she would incorporate new skills into her usual activities that would be important in planning her care.

Maintaining a safe environment

Jody was interested in protecting the environment; she bought 'green' products whenever possible. She would need teaching about her own increased susceptibility to infection, about means of prevention, and about the safe disposal of syringes.

Communicating

Jody had an enquiring mind and would possibly have no difficulties in learning the new concepts associated with the management of diabetes. She might require counselling to help her adapt to her new mode of living.

Eating and drinking

This AL would provide part of the focus of the teaching plan. Jody was a vegetarian, cooking for herself in a communal kitchen. She lived on her student grant and her diet consisted of bread, beans, salads, fruit, vegetables, cheese and eggs. She said it was difficult to keep foods in the communal fridge – food often 'disappeared' – so she cycled to the shops about a mile distant two or three times a week, although she had found this tiring lately and had not bothered with much shopping. She had previously shared the catering with her boyfriend but they had split up six weeks before. Her appetite had decreased since then, so she did less cooking anyway. Actual problems of loss of weight and a change in dietary needs for foods and fluids were identified.

156

Elimination

An increase in urine output was identified as an actual problem, and dehydration as a potential problem. Jody said she was having to pass urine at least twice during the night at present. Bowel actions were regular every day with no problems.

Personal cleansing and dressing

Although independent in this activity skin and nail care would become an important focus of care.

Working and playing

Jody was in her first year at university, reading Classical Civilisations. At present she was working hard for her end-of-first-year exams. She enjoyed the cinema and theatre and took advantage of the cheap prices on campus. For exercise she walked, cycled and swam regularly. She was not a churchgoer and had no particular beliefs. She had two special friends in her department and kept in touch with a friend from schooldays. She usually went home to her parents about twice a term. Having diabetes would not necessarily change Jody's work and leisure activities but would certainly influence the way she planned and carried them out.

Expressing sexuality

Jody had no boyfriend at present, although she had been taking oral contraceptives for eighteen months. Menstruation was regular every four weeks with no problems. Her clothes were casual, she wore no make-up, and her hair and skin looked clean and healthy. Loss of libido sometimes occurs with poorly controlled diabetes: Jody would need to be aware of this but it was not identified as a potential problem at this stage.

Jody's mother planned to stay at a nearby hotel for a few days while Jody was in hospital, and immediately after discharge to give her some support because Jody would need to return to the university in view of her exams. Jody was lethargic and not particularly interested in discussing plans for her care, but the main objectives were explained to her. These would focus on monitoring her diabetes and the modification of her medically-prescribed treatment to fit into her usual routines. Special emphasis would be on teaching related to eating and drinking, urine- and blood-glucose estimations, and the administration of insulin. As diabetes is a lifelong condition it would influence every activity of living, but as there were no problems evident at this time nursing care related to most ALs was planned chiefly as advice and information to prevent complications.

NURSING CARE: ACTIVITIES OF LIVING

Teaching and counselling the patient formed the major part of nursing care: they were planned in liaison with the specialist diabetic nurse, but mainly carried out by the primary nurse on this ward. Figure 8.3 (pages 166–70) shows the nursing care plans related to teaching. The specialist nurse would continue to provide support on discharge, in liaison with community nurses. The long-term goal was for Jody to be able by discharge to manage all aspects of her care independently, competently and confidently. The short-term goals and actions planned to meet this may be seen in the teaching plan (Figure 8.3). Despite her initial lethargy, Jody proved a willing and quick learner in theoretical aspects, but a longstanding fear of injections and a fear of sudden loss of consciousness in a hypoglycaemic episode remained with her until discharge. Recognition of hyper- and hypoglycaemic states was included in the teaching.

Jody was nursed on an acute medical ward and although John was primary nurse for patients with other conditions, he was an ideal choice as a primary nurse for a young diabetic patient. He was on duty for four of Jody's five days' stay and planned to carry out as much of her teaching or counselling as possible himself, getting to know her and the needs resulting from the onset of her illness. Counselling would be described in the AL of communicating, but although teaching is also a form of communicating it would also be described under the headings of the individual activities of living with which it was primarily concerned.

Communication (counselling)

Although a specialist diabetic nurse was in post, counselling might equally have been undertaken by any nurse with suitable skills with whom the patient had formed a good relationship. In an admission of so few days there was time for short-term counselling only; if more proved to be needed it could be continued in the community on a regular basis.

John made sure Jody had the opportunity to discuss anxieties in private. Her fear of injections (see the teaching plan, Figure 8.3) took precedence over other aspects of her condition and was the focus of counselling. She was encouraged to talk about this fear and her feelings of failure related to it. Janis (1983) suggests that even one encounter with a counsellor may establish the support a patient needs to motivate adaptive behaviour and maintain self-esteem. Jody had not overcome this fear enough to self-inject by the time she was discharged, but she had started the process and appeared more positive about it, and was less frightened about the thought of trying again using a 'pen'. She might need to be referred to a psychothera-pist for aversion therapy at a later date. When situations affecting her day-to-day life arose, she would realise implications of her illness which had seemed remote before, so would continue to need practical and emotional support from family, friends, and medical and nursing staff. Other issues were dealt with by providing relevant information. John gave her specific criteria on which to base the need to get medical advice, and advised her always to carry her medical alert card, to keep her clinic appointments, and to contact the specialist diabetic nurse at any time if she felt worried. She was told about the role of the British Diabetic Association and given the address of the local branch.

Eating and drinking

All newly-diagnosed diabetic patients are referred to the nutritionist. Jody's diet was already high in fibre, which has been shown to reduce insulin requirements and glucose levels at the recommended daily intake of about 30 g (Long and Phipps 1985). She was provided with menu suggestions and a list of exchanges for a 2000 calorie diet, including a list of foods containing 10 g of glucose for quick absorption if signs of hypoglycaemia were experienced. Nursing care consisted of giving information, teaching, monitoring the amount of food she ate, and encouraging her to make her own decisions about calculating diet needs. She was also encouraged to plan a diet and an insulin regime for discharge, taking into consideration her usual routines, work and leisure activities, alcohol intake, and level of exercise.

Personal cleansing and dressing

Loss of protein and subcutaneous fat, impaired leucocyte function and poor circulation in uncontrolled diabetes tend to reduce the effectiveness of the skin as a barrier to infection as well as slowing the healing process (Long and Phipps 1985). Nursing care consisted of information-giving, to make Jody aware of her increased susceptibility to infection, and advising her on skin and foot care in particular.

Eliminating

Urine tests do not indicate when blood-glucose is too low and do not always give an accurate measurement at the time of testing. Insulin-dependent diabetics are nevertheless encouraged to test their urine daily for the presence of ketones, which may indicate that insufficient insulin is being taken to discourage fat catabolism (Tortora and Anagnostakos 1981). This formed part of John's teaching plan.

NURSING CARE: MEDICAL PRESCRIPTION

Jody was prescribed doses of a long- and short-acting insulin twice daily. While in hospital the doses were adjusted on a sliding scale until a suitable regime was established, resulting in dosage that achieved a fasting blood-glucose level of 4–7 mmol/litre. Nursing care consisted of teaching new skills related to the administration of insulin, the estimation of blood-glucose, and concepts of diabetic management related to these activities. Information about insulin storage, care of syringes and sources of supply was given.

It was planned to teach Jody to administer her insulin using a conventional syringe at first, and when the regime was firmly established to use an insulin pen for administration. This device is loaded with a cartridge pre-filled with insulin, and the required dose is selected on a dial. Injecting is simple and quicker, and may be done more discreetly in social situations. This method of injecting may be used for any insulin regime, but in trials it has been found especially helpful in multi-injection therapy, the principle of which is to provide a base level of long-acting insulin at bedtime and quick-acting insulin before meals to imitate normal physiological response (Manning 1989). This regime might be considered for Jody at a later date to fit in with her usual routines.

SUMMARY

Jody was an intelligent girl with normal physiological and psycho-social development so had usually been at the independent pole of the continuum for all ALs. A move towards the dependent pole occurred in some ALs – eating and drinking, for example – because of lack of knowledge or skills to cope with the new requirements of her illness. In seeking medical help she had started a lifelong process of modification of her usual activities and needed to learn new skills to remain independent. The aim of the medical model was to regulate the diabetes; the aim of nursing in addition, seen in the context of this nursing model, was to help Jody incorporate the new skills so that she could carry out all her ALs in a way satisfactory to her own model for living.

Although the care was planned individually it did not all take place as planned. In different circumstances this stabilising process might have taken place in the community, but the institutional environment in which Jody lived, and the fact that her family were too far away to provide psychological or practical support, made this inappropriate. The duration of the hospital stay was based partly on the response to insulin and diet therapy (that is, the blood-glucose levels), and partly on Jody's move towards independence in activities related to this. Her longstanding fear of injections, of which nursing staff were unaware at the onset, influenced the rest of her care because her need for insulin had become a basic physiological need which she was not able to meet independently. According to a hierarchical needs theory such as that proposed by Abraham Maslow (1970), Jody would not be motivated to meet her psychosocial needs while a basic physiological need remained unmet. Her primary nurse recognised that she would need help to modify her usual activities of working and leisure, that she would need to be aware of the effects of illness or stress on her condition, and that she would need knowledge about the effects of her illness on libido or possible pregnancies. However, he realised that she would not be able to cope with more until she felt confident about carrying out activities to meet her immediate needs, so he did not introduce these topics. Her care would be continued by the community nurse and in time she might also be referred to a psychotherapist for help with her aversion to injections.

EXERCISES AND ACTIVITIES

Exercise 1

Aim   To apply the principle of individuality to planning care.

Method   Work in pairs; visit shops.

Resources Information from this chapter; calculator; college timetable (see below).

Suggested time One afternoon or morning.

Jody's timetable:
  2 days: lectures 9.30 – 4.00; 1 hour 30 minutes for lunch;
  1 day: lectures 9.30 – 12.30;
  1 day: lecture 4.00 – 5.00;
  1 day: free.

1 Plan a menu to fit in with Jody's dietary needs, her college timetable and her leisure activities.

2 Write a shopping list.

3 Price the items at your nearest shopping centre. (Agree a sum to be allowed for weekly expenditure, to include sundries.)

Exercise 2

Aim To examine critically the model's suitability for the teaching of patients.

Method Individual work.

Resources Available documentation.

Suggested time Duration of patient stay on ward *or* designated time span within this.

1 Using the framework of this model, create a teaching plan for a patient in your care who needs to learn or re-learn a particular skill. Evaluate it and modify it as required.

2 List possible reasons for the fact that Jody's teaching was not wholly successful.

3 Suggest how it could have been planned and implemented differently.

Exercise 3

Aim To plan care to meet the patient's own goals for living.

Method Discussion in groups of 4–6.

Resources Paper; pens; Erikson's development theory (see activity 2 on page 107).

Suggested time   30 minutes, plus time for presentation to the whole group.

1 In a group of 4–6, with a chosen scribe, consider an acute medical ward in your hospital.

- What is the average patient age?
- What facilities are there for younger people?
- How is privacy maintained?
- Is it a mixed-sex ward?

2 Consider the special needs of the adolescent or young adult (refer to Erikson's description of this stage). How do these needs differ from those of:

- a child;
- an older adult;
- an elderly person?

3 Discuss ways that nurses can help to meet these special needs within the resources available.

4 In the whole group, a spokesperson from each small group should present the group's ideas.

Figure 8.1

PATIENT ASSESSMENT FORM	Biographical and health

Date of admission 9 June
Date of assessment 9 June   *Signature* J.Smith

Patient
Surname COLCROSS   Forename(s) JOSEPHINE ANN
~~Male~~   **Age** 19   Prefers to be
Female   **DOB** 24 January   addressed as   JODY

Usual address Sophocles House, Redbrick University, Charbridge
(HOME ADDRESS: The Hollies, Canterbury Avenue, Farminster)
Type of accommodation
Hall of residence

Others at this residence Students

Next of kin
Name Roy Colcross   Relationship Father
Address As home address (above)
             Telephone number Farminster 59876

Significant others Mother, brother, sister, friends

Occupation Student

Religious beliefs and practices C. of E. — not practising

Recent significant life crises Onset of illness. Break-up with boyfriend.

Patient's perception of current health Good up till now. Understands that she has diabetes.

Family's perception of current health Not sought

Medical information
Chicken pox and mumps as a child. Glandular fever after A-levels (last year). No known allergies.

GP
Name Dr Little
Address Redbrick Health Centre
           Telephone number Charbridge 342881

Consultant Dr Large

Discharge plans Will need continued contact with diabetic nurse. Will require autolet, syringes, gluco-stix and insulin. Out-patient appt. for 2 weeks from discharge.

Figure 8.2

PATIENT ASSESSMENT FORM		Assessment of ALs
Name JODY COLCROSS		Date of birth 24 January
Stage of care *Admission*		Date of assessment 9 June
		Signature J Smith
Activity of living	**Usual routine**	**Problems** A : Actual P : Potential
Maintaining a safe environment	Independent.	Will be more susceptible to infection (P). Lacks knowledge about safe disposal of syringes (A).
Communicating	No speech, sight, or hearing problems.	Anxiety (P). Lack of knowledge about condition (A).
Breathing	No apparent breathing problems. Does not smoke.	Increased susceptibility to chest infections (P).
Eating and drinking	Usually has good appetite. Vegetarian. Drinks wine when she can afford it.	Change in dietary needs due to diabetes (A). Lack of knowledge about diet (A).
Eliminating	No problems usually. Regular daily bowel actions. Urinary: no problems.	Passing more urine. Needs to get up x2 at night (A). Dehydration (P).
Personal cleansing and dressing	Fully independent.	Skin is more susceptible to infection, damage, and slow healing (P).
Controlling body temperature	Fully independent.	Insulin needs may be affected by pyrexia (P).
Mobilising	Fully independent.	Extra activity may increase insulin needs (P).
Working and playing	Full-time student. Theatre, cinema, swimming, walking and cycling.	Anxious about exams (A). Usual activities affected by fatigue (A).
Expressing sexuality	Clean appearance. Menstruation regular. No boyfriend.	Will require special monitoring in any future pregnancy (P).
Sleeping	Usually about 8 hours per night.	Tired all the time recently (A).
Dying		

Figure 8.3

TEACHING PLAN		
Name JODY COLCROSS		Date of birth 24 January
Stage of care		Date 9 June
		Signature J Smith

Topic   INSULIN INJECTIONS

<u>Goals/objectives</u>

Jody will be able:
1 To identify suitable sites and to understand the reason for rotation (by 11/06)
2 To self-inject (by 12/06)
3 To draw up the correct amount of insulin (by 13/06)
4 To explain details of the storage of insulin and safe disposal of syringes (by discharge).

<u>Content/activities</u>

Demonstrate suitable sites. Ask Jody to select different site each time.

10/06 Demonstrate how to give subcutaneous injection. Allow Jody to handle syringe, examine markings. Explain as necessary.

11/06 Supervise Jody self-injecting, a.m. and p.m. Help as needed.

12/06 Explain calibrations, show how to withdraw insulin from phial and to exclude air from syringe. Encourage Jody to draw up insulin with supervision, if able.

13/06 Continue to encourage self-care but do not press her if distressed.

Explain that insulin should be stored as indicated by maker's instructions. Demonstrate ways of 'immobilising' syringes before disposal.

<u>Evaluation</u>

Discusses sites, is able to select suitable one, but is very anxious about having to give injections herself. Suggested site for injection, with some encouragement. Has no difficulty in understanding workings of syringe. JS

Held syringe but could not inject self. Very distressed says she'll never cope. P.W.

No problems with preparing injection, but became too distressed to attempt self-injection. Insulin to be given by nurses to allow time for Jody to talk about fears and calm down. JS

Tearful before injection time. Insulin given by nurse. Says she will try tomorrow, but very uncertain P.W.

Figure 8.3 (continued)

Demonstrate use of pen device; allow Jody to handle it, insert cartridge and set dial.

Seems happier about pen, but not urged to self-inject. P.W.

14/06 Provide all equipment for discharge, with written instructions. Reassure her that the district nurse will visit for evening injection and continue to help.

Anxious about return to university, coping with injections, reactions of friends, and exams; glad that her mother would stay for a few days. JS

Figure 8.3 (continued)

TEACHING PLAN		
Name JODY COLCROSS	**Date of birth** 24 January	
Stage of care	**Date** 9 June	
	Signature J Smith	

Topic ESTIMATION OF BLOOD-GLUCOSE

Goals/objectives

Jody will be able:

1 To obtain blood from fingertip (by 10/06).
2 To read and record gluco-stix result (by 11/06).
3 To identify high or low blood-glucose from readings and to take, or explain how to take, appropriate action (by discharge).
4 To take responsibility for remembering to obtain blood and for recording results (by 12/06).

Content/activities	*Evaluation*
Demonstrate use of gluco-let machine. Encourage Jody to handle it and use it herself.	10/06 Nurse obtained blood before each meal; Jody was able to read results with minimum help. Says it is not so worrying as self-injecting but is reluctant to try. JS
11/06 Continue to encourage self-use. Explain analysis of readings, desirable ranges for fasting and after-meal blood-glucose. Encourage her to work out insulin doses or diet adjustments based on estimations.	Is able to work out diet/insulin adjustments in theory without difficulty. Has not obtained own samples. P.W.
12/06 Ask Jody to obtain blood and record result, without reminder, before each meal. Check that it has been done.	Has asked nurses to obtain blood each time. No pressure put on her about it, due to her distress. JS
	13/06 obtained our blood a.m. Says it wasn't too bad. Self-care continued. P.W.
	14/06 Mild hypoglycaemic episode 6a.m. Felt weak and shaky. Tested own blood, 3.5 mmol, and reported to nurse. Glass of milk given. C.M.
	Lunchtime result: 7mmol. Anxious about further attacks at home. Counselled prior to discharge. JS

168

Figure 8.3 (continued)

TEACHING PLAN			
Name JODY COLCROSS		Date of birth	24 January
Stage of care		Date	9 June
		Signature	J Smith

Topic EATING & DRINKING

Goals/objectives

Jody will be able:
1 To work out diet exchanges using the list provided (by discharge).
2 To recognize signs of hyper- and hypoglycaemia, list causes, ways to avoid these, and actions to take.
3 To understand diet rationale and to use exchanges to compensate when insufficient diet is taken.

Content/activities

Check that Jody has understood all information given. Ask her to select diet for her individual needs from menu available, from day 1. Encourage her to plan diets for 2 normal days at home.

Explain the signs of hypoglycaemia and hyperglycaemia ~~decide~~ and what they mean. Provide a list of foods providing 10 mg glucose quickly. Explain use of 'Hypostop' syrup in emergency. Ask her to plan explanation in own words to her mother or a friend, to engage their help if needed.

Evaluation

Finds choice limited for vegetarian. Not enthusiastic about home menus because appetite is poor. Is working out what she needs to eat and drink if she cannot manage a meal. JS

Has written notes of all explanations given. Is reading the literature provided and has asked for other sources of information. JS

169

Figure 8.3 (continued)

TEACHING PLAN			
Name JODY COLCROSS		Date of birth 24 January	
Stage of care		Date 9 June	
		Signature J.Smith	
Topic ELIMINATING			

Goals/objectives
Jody will be able:
1 To test her urine for glucose and ketones.
2 To explain the significance of ketone levels.

Content/activities	*Evaluation*
Demonstrate use of reagent strips and how to read results. Explain significance and action to take if ketone levels are high. Provide chart to record results. Supervise self-testing and recording.	No problems with testing or with understanding results, but needed explanation of why this test cannot replace the blood test. Says she will read about ketones in an old biology book to help her to understand it more. No increase in ketone level during admission, urine tested daily. JS

PART III

Critique of the model

CHAPTER NINE

Analysis and evaluation

The complexity and specialisation of nursing today make it more necessary than ever for the elements of nursing to be identified and understood. (Roper *et al.* 1980)

It was because of this belief that Roper, Logan and Tierney wrote *The Elements of Nursing* in which their nursing model was first presented. One decade later, theorists and scholars continue to debate these issues. Hanucharurnkul (1989) argues that there is still no single nursing paradigm to direct practice, education or research, but only a range of phenomena related to nursing which may be interpreted in many different ways. Botha (1989) defines a paradigm as a 'group commitment to a constellation of beliefs which represent a particular way of viewing the world – in this case a discipline'. Flaskerud and Halloran (1980) present four phenomena related to nursing which appear to have been accepted as a paradigm of nursing by other nursing theorists: these are the concepts of man as the recipient of nursing care, health, the environment, and nursing. Fawcett (1989) asserts that these phenomena are central concepts which together constitute a metaparadigm of nursing. She describes a metaparadigm as 'a global perspective of a discipline', and quotes the following statement of Donaldson and Crowley (1978) as the major proposition of nursing's metaparadigm because it clearly emphasises the relationship of the four concepts:

Nursing studies the wholeness or health of humans, recognising that humans are in continuous interaction with their environment.

This critical examination of the Roper–Logan–Tierney nursing model will be carried out in two stages. In the first stage the critique will be based on the metaparadigm described by Fawcett as part of

173

her proposed framework for analysis and evaluation of a conceptual model of nursing. In the second stage it will be based on evaluation of the model in practice, using the five care studies in Part II as a framework.

Fawcett's framework for analysis and evaluation

Fawcett (1989) believes that analysis of a conceptual model of nursing poses questions about the model related to the following:

1 Development of the model
  (a) Historical evolution
  (b) Nursing knowledge development
  (c) Assumptions on which model is based

2 Content of the model
  (a) The person
  (b) The environment
  (c) Health
  (d) Nursing
  (e) Relationships between the concepts
  (f) The process of nursing

3 Areas of concern
  (a) What are the areas of concern
  (b) What is the source of the concern

She asserts that evaluation is carried out by comparing the contents of the model with criteria by which to measure the clarity of the following:

1 The assumptions
2 Comprehensiveness
3 Logical sequence
4 Ability to test theory
5 Social considerations
6 Nursing knowledge

ANALYSIS

Development of the model

Historical evolution

Roper based her original research on experience of changes in nursing between 1940 and 1970 and observed the confusion related to the clinical experience required by student nurses. She also observed that the varied descriptions of nursing as 'basic', 'bedside', 'fundamental', 'technical' or 'professional' increased confusion (Roper 1976). She quotes Jourard (1964), who argues that 'terms which label nursing according to medical specialty only lead to confusion and mask something basic which all nursing shares'. Her literature search revealed that other professions had clear statements of intent holding the same meaning for each member, and recognised that this was not so in nursing (Schwartz *et al*. 1964). It was to identify 'an image of nursing' that she carried out her exploratory research, fully described in *Clinical Experience in Nurse Education* (1976) and outlined in Part I of this book. The aim was to identify nursing requirements common to all patients, whatever their medical diagnosis; it was as a result of this that the activities of daily living (ADLs) came to be indicated as the common core of nursing practice (Roper 1976, 1979).

Roper's attempt to interpret nursing according to Wilson's (1972) belief that 'disciplines are forms of thought that have a characteristic approach to appropriate questions related to the subject' led her to develop her model of nursing based on a model of living, with the patient as the subject of nursing. She identified sixteen ADLs, and 'comforting', 'preventing' and 'seeking' activities which contributed to independence in the ADLs. The ADLs were classified as essential activities, activities which enhanced the quality of life, and one activity that reflected man's mortality. The influence of Henderson's work (1969) and Maslow's theory of human needs are acknowledged. Roper (1979) agrees that the original ADLs were developed against a background of the 'human needs' concept, but emphasises the active element of the model, later to be described by Farmer (1986) as a functional approach, by describing the ADLs as behavioural manifestations of human needs.

Later, in 1976, the Roper, Logan and Tierney team was formed and the model was developed further, until its publication in *The Elements of Nursing* (1980), which incorporated the core of nursing knowledge required and the process of nursing. By this time the sixteen ADLs had become twelve activities of living (ALs) in recognition of the fact that not every activity was performed daily. The developmental aspect of the model added a new dimension. The aim of the book was to explain the model and to facilitate new nursing knowledge related to its components. *Learning to Use the Process of Nursing* (1981) explained the model within the framework of the nursing process, while *Using a Model for Nursing* (1983) described a project in which nine nurses contributed by using the model in their own areas of practice. Work on these two books acted as a catalyst for further development and refinement of the model. As a result, explication of the 'comforting', 'preventing' and 'seeking' activities was seen as superfluous and was omitted from the 1985 version of the model. Similarly 'comforting' and 'preventing' components of nursing were incorporated into the AL role, while the dependent component was renamed collectively the 'medically or other prescriptive' role.

Nursing knowledge

Roper (1976) suggested that adoption of this model would facilitate nursing knowledge and help nursing towards professional status by developing cognitive skills and perception, quoting Tyler (1952) who asserts that intellectual operations differentiate a profession from a skilled trade. Roper envisaged the model being used as a care plan for individual care and as a structure for a nursing curriculum, in which theory related to each AL would be taught within the framework of health (Roper 1976, 1979). The model has been widely adopted in education and practice in the United Kingdom. *Principles of Nursing* (4th edition, Roper 1988), which includes aspects of most of the activities of living, surprisingly does not make this explicit as a component of the model.

Assumptions

The model makes the following assumptions:

1 The activities of living are behavioural manifestations of basic human needs common to all individuals.
2 A dependence–independence continuum, on which movement can be in either direction, is related to an individual's life span.
3 The activities of living form the core of nursing requirements.
4 The dependence–independence status of an individual in each AL is influenced by physical, psychological, sociocultural, environmental and politico-economic factors.

Content of the model

Concepts of the metaparadigm

The way in which each of the concepts of the metaparadigm has been defined in the model is examined below. It is difficult to find explicit statements about all the concepts but analysis of the literature facilitates interpretation. (See also Part I of this book.)

The person receiving the nursing care   The person receiving nursing care is seen as engaging in a process of living composed of twelve living activities through a life span from conception to death. A person's position on the life span influences the way in which the ALs are performed. A dependence–independence continuum, related to the life span, is also identified: this acknowledges changes in the dependence status for each individual in any activity of living at different times. Individuality is demonstrated by the way a person carrries out the ALs and the model recognises internal and external factors which also influence the individual performance of each AL, emphasising the uniqueness of man.

As a reminder, the ALs identified are:

- maintaining a safe environment;
- communicating;
- breathing;
- eating and drinking;
- eliminating;
- personal cleansing and dressing;
- controlling body temperature;
- mobilising;
- working and playing;
- expressing sexuality;
- sleeping;
- dying.

The interrelatedness of the activities of living and their relationship with other components of the model is accentuated throughout the model literature.

Environment   The authors make repeated references to the environment in relation to its influence on each activity of living. The focus on the ALs is intended to illustrate the individuality of each person, so it could be said that the environment is defined only in the context of its effect on the individual. In doing so the authors describe the environment as the physical, psychological, sociocultural, environmental, and politico-economic factors which influence the activities of living. They make no distinction between internal and external environment, but it may be construed that the internal environment is reflected in the description of the physiological and psychological

177

factors that influence each AL. They describe physiological influences as:

- congenital or acquired disability;
- degenerative or pathological tissue change;
- accident;
- infection.

Health The authors contend that most people see no clear distinction between health and ill health, quoting the Office of Health Economics (1971) monograph:

> It is not possible to demonstrate a cut-off point between an individual's healthy state and diseased state.

They assert that health is an individual subjective judgement and can be defined only

> in relation to the individual and his expectations and in relation to his functioning in everyday living.   (Roper *et al.* 1985)

This, however, is not an explicit statement of the model's concept of health, but demonstrates the premise on which their definition may be founded. They also comment on the widespread opinion that health takes into consideration the individual's ability to cope with and adapt to different challenges in life and the increased awareness of the potential for self-care. To reflect the notion of individuality in the model, health may be expressed as:

> The ability of a person to meet his needs by performing each activity of living in a manner acceptable to the individual, the society and the culture within which he lives, without causing harm to himself, others or the environment, according to current knowledge or beliefs. It also includes the individual successfully adapting to changes in dependence as they occur.

Nursing In contrast to the concepts of health and environment, the concept of nursing has been defined and redefined as the model has developed. This is also described in Part I of this book. Roper (1976) included in the context of a health-care system notions of activities of daily living, dependence and death when she expressed this concept in this way:

> Within the context of a health-care system and in a variety of combinations nursing is helping a person towards his personal independent pole of the continuum of each Activity of Daily Living;

helping him to remain there; helping him to cope with any movement towards the dependent poles; in some instances encouraging him to move towards the dependent pole or poles; and because man is finite, helping him to die with dignity.

A later version includes identification of different components of nursing, co-ordination of care with other disciplines, and the dimension of self-care. It was expressed thus:

> Nursing is directly or indirectly enabling each person in a health-care system to acquire, maintain or restore his maximum level of self-care/independence; or to cope with being dependent in any of his Activities of Daily Living. Nursing incorporates co-ordination of help from other health-care professions and at patient level it entails the performance of nursing activities from one or more of four groups of components of nursing. (Roper 1979)

Roper *et al.* (1985) refer to the role of the nurse in maintaining health, preventing sickness, encouraging self-help and promoting optimum independence. They maintain that the role of the nurse is dependent on a clear distinction existing between health and illness and on the fluctuating demands of society. Despite the avowed lack of distinction between health and ill health (Roper *et al.* 1985) the authors provide a clear definition of the nurse's role, focusing on the ALs as central to the role of nursing. This later statement defines nursing as helping patients to prevent, solve, alleviate or cope with actual or potential problems related to the activities of living. They attribute problems to changes in environment, routine, dependence or independence, ways of performing an AL, or discomfort associated with an AL. This role is nurse-initiated and classified as the AL component of the nursing role, an essential feature of the model. The authors also describe nurses acting in a medically or other prescriptive role when carrying out the care prescribed by doctors or other health professionals. This definition of the role of the nurse emphasises her role in the team concerned with health and health education as well as her being concerned with illness (Roper *et al.* 1985).

The process of nursing

Throughout earlier chapters of this book, the model has been described and applied in the framework of the nursing process. The authors incorporate it into their model because the process of nursing 'is neither a model nor a philosophy ... but simply a method and it needs to be used with an explicit nursing model'. They describe the nursing process as a systematic approach to patient care which helps to accomplish individualised nursing, which in the model is derived from the individuality component in the model for living (Roper *et al*. 1985). Each stage of the process is described by a verb, emphasising that the active and continuous elements in nursing correspond to the active element in the model for living characterised by ALs. 'Assessing' helps to establish previous routines, levels of independence, discomforts and problems related to each AL. 'Planning' consists of identifying interventions that will prevent potential problems becoming actual, that will solve the patient's problems, that will alleviate those that cannot be solved, or that will help the patient to cope with those that cannot be solved or alleviated. Planning includes goal-setting: in terms of the model, nursing goals must reflect the patient's own goals for living and must indicate the desired behaviour in each AL. 'Implementing' the nursing care may be derived from problems in an AL or from medical or other professional prescription. 'Evaluating' is a means of establishing whether the goals have been achieved and involves comparing the actual behaviour in each AL with the desired behaviour stated in the goal.

The relationship between the concepts

The relationship between the concepts of health and man is demonstrated by the statement that

> health can be defined only in relation to the individual and his expectations, and in relation to his optimum level of functioning in everyday living. (Roper *et al*. 1985)

If health is conceptualised thus, the 1979 and 1985 definitions of nursing (above) also illustrate the relationship between man, nursing and health.

The assertion that the definition of nursing relies on the clear distinction between health and ill health (Roper *et al*. 1985) may be construed in itself as a demonstration of the relationship of the concepts of health and nursing in this model. Any definition of nursing based on this premise must implicitly illustrate this relationship.

The latest definition of nursing in the model (1985) explains the relationships between nursing, man and the environment by identifying environmental factors as a cause of problems related to ALs, which nursing is trying to alleviate, prevent or solve. However the concepts of health and environment remain implicit rather than explicit.

Areas of concern This model focuses on the ability of the individual to perform the activities of living. The source of the problem is seen as any factor that influences the dependence–independence status of the individual in any activity of living.

EVALUATION

Clarity of the assumptions

Evaluation examines the way in which the assumptions are explained and the nature of the values expressed in the model. Roper attempts to clarify the assumption that the ALs are behavioural manifestations of human needs by using the fourteen basic human needs identified by Henderson (1969), and later adopted by the International Council for Nurses, as a source for her original list of ADLs. She categorised these in a way similar to that of Maslow (1954) as those that are essential for life and those that enhance the quality of life. She also added dying to this list, to represent man's mortality. The assumption that dependence and independence is related to a person's life span has been explained by reference to life-span development theories, such as that proposed by Erikson (1950) and by description of the factors that influence the dependence status of an individual. However the model does not indicate a means of measuring the level of dependence in any AL, which would facilitate goal-setting and evaluation of nursing care. The assumption that the ALs form the core of nursing care was developed as a result of inductive reasoning which led to exploratory research. It has been fully explained in the literature since the model's inception (Roper 1976, 1979; Roper et al. 1980, 1985). The fourth assumption, which identifies the factors that influence dependence or independence in each AL, may be observed empirically.

Great value is placed in the model on individuality: it is identified as a component of the model for living which in turn is reflected in individual nursing care. Value is also placed on observable behaviour as an indication of the *need* for nursing and the basis of evaluation of the *effects* of nursing.

181

Comprehensiveness of the concepts

The authors' definition of the person receiving the care is comprehensive and has developed from scientific theory from the biological, psychological and social sciences. The concept of health is not clearly defined but is seen as a subjective state for each individual. This may be seen as the premise on which this nursing model is based. If the goal of nursing is health or wholeness (however this is defined), then nursing care based on the patient's model for living will aim to achieve the state of health for that individual as he himself subjectively experiences it. Although the environment is never explicitly defined as a concept, it is repeatedly referred to in the model literature and environmental factors which influence the ALs are described comprehensively. The authors focus on the external environment; and although physical and psychological influences are recognised, they are not explicitly defined as the internal environment. Similarly, the social, cultural, economic and political influences are described, but not within the parameters of the environment. Like the concept of man, nursing is clearly defined. The definitions have been expanded as the model has developed, demonstrating a degree of pragmatism in the dynamic approach. Nursing is described within the context of health care, emphasising the role of health and illness, and the relationship of the nurse's role to those of other health professionals.

Evaluation of the 'nursing process' component of the model in Fawcett's framework is based on five criteria proposed by Walker and Nicholson (1989). They say that the nursing process should:

- incorporate a knowledge base;
- permit dynamic movement between the stages;
- be applicable to nursing in general;
- be compatible with ethical standards;
- be consistent with scientific findings related to human behaviour.

Does the Roper–Logan–Tierney model meet these criteria? First, it does incorporate a knowledge base for the twelve ALs which represent the core of nursing practice. This includes knowledge of the nature and purpose of each AL and of the associated body structure and function required for its performance. In addition, the nurse needs knowledge of all the factors influencing the ALs and the nature of the related problems, including knowledge from the psychological and social sciences. Second, the essence of the model is action, exemplified by the use of verbs to describe the ALs and the four stages of the process of nursing. This emphasises the ongoing nature of each phase, suggesting a dynamic movement between them. This is made explicit in the model literature. Third, the applicability to nursing in general is implied by the statement that the model is deliberately broad and simple because

> we believe that ... there is – and should be – a consensus among nurses as to the beliefs, goals and practices which are common to nursing, whatever the particular setting or circumstances, disease condition or patient/client group involved. (Roper *et al.* 1985)

Applicability has also been demonstrated in a very small way by using the model in nine different settings, as described in *Using a Model for Nursing* (Roper *et al.* 1983). However, although one of the settings was concerned with health visiting, Clark (1986) suggests that a model conceptualising the recipient of care as an individual person and focusing on problems cannot be applied to health visiting. Pearson (1983) describes its application in a clinical nursing unit, while Wright (1986) acknowledges its relevance in creating his own model of nursing in an elderly care unit. Adoption in the United Kingdom in both practice and education has been widespread. Fourth, compatibility with ethical standards is shown by the emphasis on the individual's right to self-determination, illustrated by the fact that the model of nursing follows the patient's model for living, and also by the recognition of an individual's subjective perception of his own state of well-being. Finally, the model uses scientific findings related to human behaviour to explain the ALs, consistent with the fifth criterion.

Logical sequence

This aspect of evaluation concerns what are described by Fawcett (1989) as 'world views' of 'mechanism' or 'organicism', 'change' or 'persistence'. The mechanistic view is that a person is inherently passive and reacts to external forces, while the organismic view suggests that a person is an integrated, organised entity, spontaneously active and interacting with the environment, and that behaviour is related to structural changes in the person. The view of change focuses on growth whereas the opposite view, of persistence, focuses on stability (Fawcett 1989). The Roper–Logan–Tierney model appears to reflect the organismic view. They describe the person as an active being and the interrelationship of the ALs suggests holism. Changes in dependence status may occur as a result of structural changes related to the ALs. Conversely, the assumption that man is influenced by the environment suggests the passivity outlined in the mechanistic view. The view of change is demonstrated in the model in the bidirectional movement on the dependence–independence continuum and in growth through the developmental phases inherent in the life span. 'As a person moves along the life span there is continuous change' (Roper *et al*. 1985). However, it could be argued that stability is the desired state and nursing is aiming to restore stability by focusing on regaining or maintaining independence in each AL.

Ability to test theory

The model has been described as a systems model (Aggleton and Chalmers 1987), as an eclectic model incorporating multiple theories (Thibodeau 1983) and as an 'activities of living' model based on human needs (McFarlane 1980); Farmer (1986) describes it as having a functional approach. Pearson (1983) describes it as a systems/development-based model incorporating concepts of Orem's model and the conceptual framework of Henderson's model. Roper *et al*. (1986) do not intend their model to be primarily a theoretical construction but see it as an intermediate stage in theory development. However, there is an indication that historically Roper used inductive reasoning to develop her model (as described earlier in this chapter). The interdependence of the ALs suggests the theoretical foundation of systems theory. The systems theory characteristic of internal and external stress is illustrated by identification of factors influencing the ALs. Homeostasis is discussed in relation to the physiology of the ALs, but a state of equilibrium in other ALs is assumed rather than defined, nor is feedback clarified.

The notion that the twelve ALs are behavioural manifestations of human needs, based on Henderson's list of basic human needs, illustrates this theoretical orientation. The hierarchical and motivational aspects of human-needs theory, which proposes that the individual must meet basic needs before he is motivated to meet the higher needs for love, self-esteem and self-actualisation, are not clear in the model. Minshull *et al*. (1986) criticise the over-simplification of this concept and the emphasis on biological needs in the model. However, Roper *et al*. do not claim that the model reflects all aspects of human needs but only that it was developed against a background of human-needs theory (Roper 1979; Roper *et al*. 1983a).

Characteristics of development theory are evident in the life-span component of the model. The authors address the developmental aspect of dying, which is sometimes ignored in this theory, where an increased value must be attached to each stage of development. They comment on the stages of grieving proposed by Kubler-Ross (1969), described as denial, isolation, anger, bargaining and depression. They do not include a stage of acceptance but in quoting Cassons (1980) – 'dying makes life suddenly real ... it has been the greatest adventure of my life' – they emphasise the 'value' placed on this stage. Although identifiable stages on the life span are discussed, the distinctions are not made clear in relation to the model for nursing and identifiable tasks for each stage are not clarified.

Some perspectives of this model pose questions which may generate theory-testing. Pain is described by the authors as a complex phenomenon, with physiological, psychological and socio-cultural aspects, which is the subject of considerable research. If it is not clearly related to a specific AL, they suggest that it be included for the purposes of nursing care under the AL of communication (Roper *et al.* 1985). Further research may be required to establish the extent to which this is appropriate. The assumption that ALs are influenced by external factors could be tested by examining the differences or similarities in dependence–independence status in a particular AL for people in different socioeconomic or cultural groups. Use of the continuum to assess patient dependence in order to establish nursing levels might also be explored.

Social considerations

Expectations

Roper, Logan and Tierney base their model on a model for living, and the goals of nursing should therefore reflect the individual's goals for living. Because it identifies the social and cultural influences on the ALs the model links not only with the expectations of the individual but also with those of society. However the notion of independence in carrying out ALs may not always be congruent with the expectations of patients, some of whom may find difficulty in relinquishing the dependent patient role.

Social significance and utility

Results of the study concerned with using the model to nurse nine patients in different care settings revealed that all patients and families were positive about the nurse–patient relationship established when using the model. Recognising potential problems encouraged nurses to provide more information and teaching, and assessing 'the whole person' induced a welcoming feeling for patients. In terms of social utility, Roper (1976) suggested use of the model in education and curriculum development, which has now become reality in a great number of nurse education centres. She also proposes its use as a means of rating patient dependency in each AL to provide quantitative data as a basis for research. This could also provide administrative information.

In addition to the descriptions by Pearson and Wright, whose work is described above, application in paediatrics is described in three papers. Wilding *et al.* (1988) outline the advantages of using the ALs for assessment of babies in a neonatal unit; Clark and Bishop (1988) discuss their own eclectic model based on this model and on Orem's in a children's hospital; and a similar undertaking by Clark (1988) describes the construction of their developmental/ behavioural paediatric model of nursing using activities of living from the Roper–Logan–Tierney model with the addition of two of their own. Application of the model within a computerised Hospital Information System is described in the Appendix.

Contribution to nursing knowledge

The 'activities of living' framework of this model provides an explicit focus for nursing assessment and actions. The emphasis on independence and individual perception of health goals encourages patient-centred nursing and is relevant to current views of health care. The incorporation of the process of nursing provides a systematic approach, and the vocabulary used in the model is easily understood by nurses in Britain, thereby avoiding confusion in interpretation and practice.

EVALUATING THE MODEL IN PRACTICE

Roper, Logan and Tierney state that their model is intended to provide an overall framework in which to practise the process of nursing. It is deliberately broad to permit flexibility; nurses are encouraged to apply it to any area of practice. With the exception of breathing, the authors suggest no priority in the ALs because the priority for each individual will differ according to circumstances. They overcome part of the difficulty of classifying problems by including the component of care derived from medical or other prescription, which helps to prevent the awkwardness of trying to make every problem conform to the AL framework (Roper *et al.* 1985). The real test of any model, however, is how it works in practice. The questions we must ask when attempting to evaluate the use of a model are these:

1 Does the model help the nurse to assess the patient thoroughly?
2 Does the information collected help to make a nursing diagnosis? Does it then help in identifying the problems that are amenable to nursing intervention?
3 Does the model facilitate goal-setting?
4 Are appropriate nursing interventions suggested by the use of this model?
5 What criteria are suggested for the evaluation of nursing care based on the use of the model?

This part of the chapter will focus on the phases of the process of nursing and the nurse's role as applied to the five care studies presented in Part II of this book.

Assessing

The ALs provided a good framework for assessing in all five care studies, helping to build up a composite picture of the patient as a whole person, and his or her family when relevant. The questions posed by assessing in the individuality component of the model (such as how, how often, why and when) furnished information not only about the way in which the person carried out each AL but also the knowledge and beliefs he or she held about it; recognition of the factors influencing the ALs facilitated understanding about this. For example, in Chapter 4 Margaret's assessment showed that she expressed her femininity by the way she dressed and cared for herself, but she was also at the post-menopausal stage where many women experience a change in body image and lose confidence in their sexual attractiveness: this would be a major influence on the way she would adapt to a further change of body image after surgery. James Matthews, the subject of the care study in Chapter 5, was seen from the assessment as a dedicated professional, putting his parish work before his own needs, which influenced the way in which he carried out many of his ALs: this information provided a basis for suggesting changes in his lifestyle after his heart attack. In Chapter 6 the information about George's usual routines, his favourite toys and his vocabulary, combined with knowledge related to his stage of development, helped nurses to plan his care in order to cause minimal disruption in his life. Annie, in Chapter 7, emerged as a lady rather set in her ways, doing the same thing at the same time every day. This is comprehensible when seen in the context of her social circumstances, having lived in the same house for so many years and never working outside the home. This made it easier to understand why she did not adapt readily to the changes imposed by her limited mobility after discharge. In the final care study, Jody's dietary and insulin needs were established within the framework of her usual working and leisure routine, to take into account her vegetarianism and the financial constraints upon her.

Identification of problems

The lack of rigidity related to priority among the ALs allows the nurse to decide individual priorities for each patient. It will be seen how this was reflected in the care studies. Problems related to eliminating and eating and drinking were seen as priorities in Margaret's immediate pre-operative care, and because she was anxious about sleeping this also assumed more importance than other ALs. Immediately after the operation, breathing became the priority while later her altered body image caused sexuality to be considered. Pain and anxiety were major problems for James Matthews, making communicating a priority, although a shift towards working and playing occurred as he approached discharge. In George's case (with the exception of the immediate post-op. period) the unfamiliar people and language, and the change in his usual routine, made communicating and playing priorities throughout his stay. For Annie, mobilising provided the major focus throughout most of her first admission and at home; breathing and controlling body temperature were the focus of the second admission. In Jody's care the interrelatedness of the ALs is illustrated to the extent that no single AL emerges as a clear priority.

Despite clear guidelines given by the model, there do appear to be some difficulties in categorising some problems in practice. The problem of pain was identified in *Using a Model for Nursing* (1983), and was resolved to some extent by addressing pain not specifically related to an AL under the heading of communicating. This is logically explained, as pain is subjective and can be identified by a nurse by the way in which it is communicated. In the case of James Matthews, this seemed entirely appropriate: his pain and anxiety were major problems, communicated both verbally and non-verbally, and needing immediate attention. Conversely Annie's pain was associated with mobilising so categorisation was clearly indicated. It is classification of problems related to nursing interventions that appears to be more uncertain; these are discussed later.

Setting goals and planning care

The emphasis in this model is on nursing encouraging patients to achieve, maintain or regain their maximum independence or to help them adapt to dependence. Assessing an individual's dependence in each AL and judging to what extent nursing will be able to promote movement on the dependence–independence continuum provide the foundation for setting goals and planning care (Roper *et al.* 1985). The deliberate breadth of the model allows nurses to agree their own goals within the framework, but the breadth may also militate against having clearly stated objectives. There has to be some consensus about levels of dependence in each AL if all nurses are to share the same meaning about a patient. Individuality is observed in relation to the way in which each AL is performed and in the factors that influence it at each level of dependence. This deficit – or by implication flexibility – of the model is most clearly illustrated by the study of Annie, in which nurses had devised their own guide for assessing on the continuum.

Goals in terms of this model should also reflect the patient's own goals for living – the emphasis is on the partnership in care. Differences in perception between patient and nurse may cause difficulties in interpretation: the patient's goals may be considered unsuitable by the nurse in the context of current beliefs about health or values placed on self-care. The fact that Margaret did not wish her husband to see her stoma while the nurse thought this would be an indication of acceptance of body image reflects this dichotomy. It also illustrates the fact that the time span within which the nurse and patient expected the goal to be achieved may have been unrealistic. Following nursing care in hospital, the patient and her partner may have continued to try to meet this goal at home, which demonstrates the nurse's responsibility in continuity of care.

All five care studies included goals set to prevent potential problems from becoming actual problems, which illustrates the preventive aspect of the nurse's role in this model.

Implementing the nursing plan

Nursing care may be derived from ALs or from medical and other prescription. Both aspects have been demonstrated in the five care studies, and although there does not always appear to be a clear

189

distinction between the two components, such a distinction would be mainly academic. For example, much pre-operative care is medically prescribed but directly related to a specific AL. Preparation of the bowel is related to elimination; skin preparation to personal cleansing and dressing; 'nil by mouth' to the activities of eating and drinking. The same principle may be applied to immediate care following operation or medical emergency. Haemorrhage, for example, is considered for physiological reasons in the activity of breathing, yet as it could occur from any part of the body it could instead be related to specific ALs: the classification may be different in each situation and will not concern busy nurses as they carry out the care. Similarly, to assess unconsciousness with sleep may seem physiologically sound but in terms of nursing care it is the activities affected by the unconscious state, such as breathing, which concern nurses. For this reason, no clear stance has been taken in these studies, and in my own opinion the categorising of nursing care should assume importance only in relation to directing thinking and practice towards providing a high quality of nursing care.

Nursing actions are planned to help achieve goals, as described above, but the model does not always direct the organisation of care or selection of appropriate interventions needed to motivate patients to reach their goals. This is particularly so in the case of James Matthews's spiritual distress. Spirituality is not addressed in the model, except in terms of the influence of religion and culture on individual activities. Mr Matthews was fortunate in having a spiritual mentor: as nursing has a 24-hour responsibility, how are *nurses* guided to act in problems such as this? The life-span component is useful in identifying the developmental stage of the patient but not always its significance to nursing care. In Chapter 6, nursing care was based on knowledge of George's developmental stage, but descriptions of only a few ALs included reference to appropriate nursing actions; the relevance of cognitive development in language was not expanded enough to make a significant difference to the way he was nursed. The role of the nurse in teaching is mentioned in relation to breathing, self-medication, safety, hygiene, working and playing, and stoma care, but as an overall component in nursing it is implicit rather than explicit. The teaching in Chapter 8 was not totally successful. The lack of a definition of motivation in the concept of the person receiving the care may have contributed to this. Lewis (1988) considers that the model ignores pathophysiology when the real emphasis on a surgical ward is on unstable physiology. Tierney (1984) comments on this and discusses the planned alterations. The redefinition of the medically-prescribed component of nursing in the 1985 version and the description of the pathophysiological influences on the ALs included from the model's inception partially address this criticism.

Evaluating

The purpose of evaluation is to establish to what extent the goals have been met. It cannot be stressed enough that it can only be carried out effectively if the goals are explicit. The continuum and the recognition of individuality allow for clear goal-setting to provide criteria for evaluation. The dynamic nature of the model is illustrated by setting new goals when existing ones are met, at a stage further along the continuum, and the principle that the nursing should reflect the patient's own model for living encourages the participation of the patient in evaluation. The positive and negative aspects of each stage of the process also influence evaluating; this will occur whichever model is used. Within these constraints the Roper–Logan–Tierney model provides clear guidelines for evaluating and expresses the dynamic nature of the nursing process.

SUMMARY

Many readers may question the necessity of evaluating a model of nursing – essentially a practical activity – in a theoretical framework. However, as demonstrated in Part I of this book, theory and practice are inextricably linked so that a model that does not clarify its theoretical concepts may not clarify its relevance to practice. For this purpose both theoretical and practical perspectives have been addressed in this critique.

From the analysis and evaluation carried out within Fawcett's framework, it may be seen that the model has been developed and expanded since its inception and has been widely adopted by education and practice. Concepts of the person and nursing are comprehensively defined and described, reflecting the model's development, while the concepts of health and environment receive extensive mention and are clarified by analysis of the model literature. The relationship of the concepts is incorporated in the definitions and in part by the diagrammatic representation of the Roper–Logan–Tierney model (Roper *et al.* 1985, p. 64). The assumptions are stated clearly and explained in terms of existing theory, exploratory research and empirical observation. The process of nursing incorporated in the model appears to meet four of the five criteria proposed by Walker and Nicholson. The fifth, applicability to nursing, is claimed by the authors (Roper *et al.* 1983, 1985) but challenged by authors such as Clark and Lewis (above). The model's stance in terms of mechanism versus organicism and change versus persistence appears to be ambivalent. The theoretical orientation is eclectic and poses questions for further research. The model is based on an individual's model for living, and thus represents some of society's current health expectations. The activities of living provide a systematic approach encouraging individual patient care, and the model is articulated in language familiar to nurses in Britain. This model appears to meet many but not all of the criteria for a theoretical model, as would be expected: it has never been described as such by the authors, who see it as a stage in theory development:

A model is an artefact, it provides growing points for new ideas.

(Roper *et al.* 1983)

Aggleton and Chalmers (1987) explore the usefulness of a nursing model in the framework of the nursing process and concepts of man and nursing role. This is the basis of the method used to evaluate the five care studies in the present work. Jackson (1986) states that

A model is not a recipe book. If used as such it would lead to a different form of ritualistic care.

Roper *et al.* (1985) agree and argue in favour of their model being broad and simple by claiming that a model does not need to exhaust every aspect of the subject. This principle helps to avoid ritualistic care, although the lack of suggestions as a foundation for appropriate interventions has been identified. Jackson adds that a model must cover diverse situations, make a positive difference to a patient's care, and encourage nurses to work as a unified team. In this book the model has been applied to patients in different situations and evaluation has affirmed the existence of a positive influence on patient care. It also attests the assertion of Meleis (1985) that a model should make nursing more effective by providing a guide to assessment and goal-setting, an explanation of nursing actions and criteria by which to evaluate outcomes.

In conclusion, this model is articulated in a way that nurses understand. The 'activities of living' component is useful and logical for nurses to apply to the stages of the nursing process and encourages consideration of the 'whole person' approach. The continuum puts a value on self-care as a goal of health and facilitates the evaluation of care, while the introduction of a life-span approach emphasises the developmental aspects of care, especially for children and the elderly. McFarlane (1986) believes that nursing models based on ideas which are not derived from practice will seem unreal and lack usefulness. Pearson (1983) encapsulates this when he says:

Real nurses nursing real patients are busy and tired, and therefore unable to engage in eleborate conceptual exercises throughout their working day.

The Roper–Logan–Tierney model is based on ideas derived from practice and may be seen to be useful in practice – for real nurses, nursing real people.

Automated care planning

The lady with the lamp has become the professional with the terminal, the cool hand on the fevered brow a hand operating the keyboard.

Van Bemmel, J. H. 1987. Computer-assisted care in nursing.
In *Computers in Nursing*, 5(4), July/August.

In April 1989, automated patient-care planning was introduced in three wards at The Royal Hampshire County Hospital (RHCH), Winchester. By November of the same year, sixteen wards were using the new system. This progress resulted from much work and repeated modification of the system. The description below does not include the problems and difficulties, which do exist; neither does it include the ongoing alteration and modification, because space does not allow this. Brief descriptions are given of the background to the system, the decision-making process and the change process; and an example of an existing care plan is included even though this plan is even now being ruthlessly changed. Current modification aims to produce more succinct care plans with the care planning standards on 'help' screens for reference and guidance only. To discuss these developments would take another book! The assessments and care plans are based on the Roper–Logan–Tierney model and are part of the automated Hospital Information System established as a component of the Wessex Regional Information Systems Plan (RISP).

How it all started

RISP is a policy on information and information systems, drawn up in consultation with District Health Authority representatives. It is an integrated information system, established in order to devise the best way of utilising resources to meet the increased demand for services, by enabling more cost-effective clinical and managerial decisions.

The system has five core systems, of which Hospital Services is one. This is subdivided into four functional components, including Patient Care in which care planning is a function. Implementation of Hospital Services (HIS) was planned in three phases. Phase 1 includes Patient Administration; Phase 2, Patient Care functions; and Phase 3, Out-Patient Clinics.

Software

Wessex Regional Health Authority selected TDS (formerly Technicon) as a software supplier for the system. Having standard software throughout the region reduces the risk of incompatibilities or difficulties which may be experienced when using multiple systems. It also facilitates user familiarity.

Education and training for the new system

Education for Phase 1 of the implementation process was organised by the TDS team. Additional trainers were selected from hospital staff and given two days' intensive training prior to the start of the training programme. All staff were required to attend a compulsory introductory session and other components relevant to their roles. Personal identification numbers (PINs) with which to gain access to the system were issued on completion of the relevant components. Different grades of staff were allocated different areas of access as appropriate. Training and allocation of PINs is now part of the orientation programme for new staff.

Decisions related to patient care planning

A Care-Planning Sub-Committee was established to choose the nursing model, the care-planning terminology, and pathways to access care-planning information. Representatives included members from TDS, nurse education and practice from the RHCH, and two other districts. Information was passed to the nurse user-group, made up of nurses representing each clinical unit, so that information could be distributed to all the wards.

PATIENT CARE PLANS

The terms selected for use in care planning are 'assessment', 'goals', 'actions', 'evaluation' and 'progress notes'. The Roper–Logan–Tierney model of nursing was chosen because it was an established part of the nursing curriculum in nurse education. Although nurses were familiar with the 'activities of living' component of the model it had not been made explicit in the paper documentation, so that there was little evidence to identify use of the model in practice. Automating the care plans provided the opportunity to make model-based practice more explicit.

Three pathways by which to access care plans were established.

Activity of living Problems affecting ALs are categorised under the heading of each activity.

Speciality The care plans reflect the way in which the medical component of nursing care affects each activity of living.

Free type Pathways and headings were provided so that nurses can create their own care plans.

To preserve individuality and flexibility each care plan may be created using a single pathway or a combination of pathways, and may have additional 'free type' problems attached.

THE NURSING PROCESS

Assessment

Three different assessments are available: adult; paediatric; and day surgery.

Following hospital policy that patients staying less than 72 hours do not *necessarily* require a full assessment, the adult assessment indicates the elements which are required for *all* patients, allowing nurses to use their professional judgement in the case of short-stay patients. The assessment screens provide a pro forma for general information and clinical observations, and (with the exception of day surgery) for assessing ALs. For each AL there are pre-written statements related to the individual way in which ALs are performed: these may be selected by light pen. In addition, the 'free type' facility allows extra information to be included. Use of the

Norton scale to assess pressure-sore vulnerability is included in the AL of personal cleansing and dressing. A 'key point' summary at the end allows problem identification based on the assessment.

Problem statements

The problems are derived from ALs or from medically or other initiated prescriptions: they are patient-orientated. As far as possible they are expressed to reflect the way in which the patient experiences the problem. Nurses may add to each problem statement using free type.

Setting goals

Goal statements include measurable and observable criteria by which to evaluate where appropriate, reflecting the model's assumption that ALs are behavioural manifestations of human needs. Each goal may be light-pen selected; a facility for adding a goal date allows the nurse to judge when there is likely to be an observable change which may be evaluated. Each goal may be individualised by use of free type, or whole goals may be free-typed and included in the care plan.

Planning the nursing actions

Each action statement includes specific details about the time, method and resources for carrying out the care, where appropriate. (This is less easy when actions relate to emotional care.) Actions are light-pen selectable and may be individualised in the same way as the goals.

Evaluating

Evaluation is goal-orientated and there are several ways to carry it out. If a goal is achieved, it may be 'completed' by selecting a statement to that effect. If the relevant action is no longer required, that may be 'completed' by the same means. Similarly a whole problem may be resolved. However, if a goal is *not* achieved, a selection of appropriate statements is available to provide a rationale, and there is a facility to write a new date for evaluation. To comply with the dynamic aspect of the process, new goals and actions may be added at any time.

Progress notes

This pathway allows nurses to free-type any information which they feel does not logically fit into care planning.

OPERATING AUTOMATED CARE PLANNING

Collecting the data for care planning

The 'nursing process' approach to patient care has been used at the RHCH since 1980, so it is a familiar method of organisation. Major change may be very stressful: in an attempt to minimise the stress, nurses were involved in planning the content of the new care plans so that they would be familiar with this aspect, if not the technological aspects, of care planning. Each of the sixteen wards identified one or two nurses who provided all the information usually included in care planning on the ward. The way in which this was produced was decided by the nurses: in some cases it was verbal, given during interviews, in others it was listed or written in a care-plan form. The information was collated and care-plan statements were written by nurses in the Research and Development department, using the principles of the Roper–Logan–Tierney model. These were submitted to the ward for approval (on paper) and were modified if necessary. Since implementation further minor modifications have been carried out as required.

HIS project team

This team is led by a senior nurse. The nursing section has a lead nurse analyst and two supporting nurse analysts who are trained in the use of TDS tools, in order to develop screens and create output documents (such as those required for assessment and care planning). The care-planning screens were designed in such a way that nurses in the Research and Development team who wrote the care plans are able to type them in and carry out modifications themselves.

Education and support for automated care planning

Designated nurses from each unit were taken from the clinical area for a period of time to train nurses in the use of the care-plan pathways. They were prepared for this role by nurse members of the

HIS project team, who provided 24-hour support to the wards during the implementation phase. On average, ward nurses had a full day's formal training, with further individual tuition as required. This tuition is now included in the orientation programme for new nurses. The computer-based training programme is also used for students during training.

Future plans

Work continues on the care plans. Modifications are based on constant feedback from the users and on information obtained from an ongoing audit programme carried out by the Research and Development group. At present a pilot study is being planned to incorporate and evaluate further changes, involving more explicit use of standard statements within care planning.

SUMMARY

This short description has aimed to present a brief overview of the application of this nursing model in an automated system for care planning. It has not attempted to be analytical in any way, or to identify strengths or weaknesses. It is not intended to be a comprehensive description of the system in the context of Hospital Information Systems.

Figure A.1 *Example of computer care plan*

```
ACTIVITY OF LIVING: COMMUNICATING

PROBLEM
Anxiety caused by unfamiliar environment,
routine and terminology.

GOALS
* To feel comfortable in new routine with
  no sense of isolation.
* To demonstrate understanding of condition
  and treatment by explaining in own words.
* To be able to identify relevant
  personnel.
```

```
*  To be able to locate own bed area and
   ward facilities as appropriate.
*  To be able to express anxieties and
   specific worries.
*  To show fewer verbal and non-verbal signs
   of anxiety.

ACTIONS
*  Introduce patient to self, other staff
   and patients.
*  Clarify name patient wishes to be
   addressed by.
*  Inform about visiting times, ward
   routines and facilities.
*  Establish present level of knowledge
   related to condition and treatment.
   Explain as necessary, using suitable
   terms.
*  Make use of diagrams, pictures in
   explanations.
*  Show round ward, clarify facilities that
   may be used.
*  Clarify safety rules about smoking.
*  Allow time and privacy to facilitate
   discussion and expression of feelings.
*  Include family members in
   discussions/explanations.
```

Figure A.2 *A care plan as selected and used, with reference to Margaret Wells (Chapter 4)*

```
ACTIVITY OF LIVING: COMMUNICATING

PROBLEM
Anxiety caused by unfamiliar environment,
routine and terminology.

GOAL 5/5 To demonstrate understanding of
condition and treatment by explaining in
own words. 5/5 Evaluation: Margaret has
good understanding of condition and stoma.
Goal achieved.[1]
```

GOAL 5/5 To be able to identify relevant personnel.

GOAL 5/5 To be able to locate own bed area and ward facilities as appropriate. 5/5 Evaluation: Goal achieved.

GOAL 5/5 To be able to express anxieties and specific worries. 6/5 Evaluation: Margaret seems anxious still but has not expressed any specific anxieties. 8/5 Evaluation: Showed distress, expressed fears about stoma in general.

GOAL 5/5 To show fewer verbal and non-verbal signs of anxiety. 8/5 Evaluation: Still rather tense.

ACTION 5/5 Introduce patient to self, other staff and patients. 5/5 Completed.

ACTION 5/5 Inform about visiting times, ward routines and facilities. 5/5 Completed.[2]

ACTION 5/5 Establish present level of knowledge related to condition and treatment. Explain as necessary, using suitable terms.

ACTION 5/5 Show round ward, clarify facilities that may be used. 5/5 Completed.

ACTION 5/5 Clarify safety rules about smoking. Explain smoking in day room only. 5/5 Completed.

ACTION 5/5 Allow time and privacy to facilitate discussion and expression of feelings.

ACTION 5/5 Include family members in discussions/explanations.

---

1 *Achieved goals will not continue to appear on the screen but may be retrieved from the system at any time during the patient's admission and for 4 weeks following discharge.*
2 *Completed actions are treated in the same way as achieved goals.*

Figure A.3 *The care plan as it will appear on the screen on 6 May*

ACTIVITY OF LIVING: COMMUNICATING

PROBLEM
Anxiety caused by unfamiliar environment,
routine and terminology.

GOAL 5/5 To be able to identify relevant
personnel.

GOAL 5/5 To be able to express anxieties
and specific worries. 6/5 Evaluation:
Margaret seems anxious still but has not
expressed any specific anxieties. 8/5
Evaluation: Showed distress, expressed
fears about stoma in general.

GOAL 5/5 To show fewer verbal and
non-verbal signs of anxiety. 8/5
Evaluation: Still rather tense.

ACTION 5/5 Establish present level of
knowledge related to condition and
treatment. Explain as necessary, using
suitable terms.

ACTION 5/5 Allow time and privacy to
facilitate discussion and expression of
feelings.

ACTION 5/5 Include family members in
discussion/explanations.

Chapter 1

Abdellah, F. G., Beland, I. L., Martin, A. and Matheny, R. V. 1960. *Patient-Centered Approaches*. New York: Macmillan.

Botha, M. E. 1989. Theory development in perspective; the role of conceptual frameworks and models in theory development. In *Journal of Advanced Nursing*, **14**, 49–55.

Chin, P. L. and Jacobs, M. K. 1983. *Theory and Nursing: a systematic approach*. St. Louis: Mosby.

Chin, R. 1980. The utility of systems and development models for practice. In Riehl and Roy 1980.

Faulkner, A. 1985. *Nursing: a creative approach*. Avon, England: Bailliere Tindall.

Flaskerud, J. H. and Halloran, E. J. 1980. Areas of agreement in nursing theory development. In *Advances in Nursing Science*, **3**(1).

George, J. (ed.) 1985. *Nursing Theory*. New Jersey: Prentice-Hall.

Hagell, E. I. 1989. Nursing knowledge women's knowledge: a sociological perspective. In *Journal of Advanced Nursing*, **14**, 226–33.

Hazzard, M. E. and Kergin, D. J. 1971. An overview of systems theory. In *Nursing Clinics of North America*, **6** (3). (Quoted in Riehl and Roy 1980.)

Hockey, L. (ed.) 1981. *Current Issues in Nursing*. Edinburgh: Churchill Livingstone.

Johnson, D. 1975. Unpublished lecture notes and class handouts. University of California at Los Angeles. (Quoted in Riehl and Roy 1980.)

Meleis, A. I. 1985. *Theoretical Nursing: development and practice*. Pennsylvania, USA: Lippincott.

Nightingale, F. 1859. *Notes on Nursing*. London: Duckworth.

Orlando, I. 1961. *The Dynamic Nurse–Patient Relationship*. New York: Putnam.

Riehl, J. P. and Roy, C. (eds) 1980. *Conceptual Models for Nursing Practice*. USA: Appleton Century-Crofts.

Roper, N. 1976. *Clinical Experience in Nurse Education.* Edinburgh: Churchill Livingstone.

Roper, N., Logan, W. and Tierney, A. 1980. *The Elements of Nursing,* 1st edn. Edinburgh: Churchill Livingstone.

Roper, N., Logan, W. and Tierney, A. 1981. *Learning to Use the Process of Nursing.* Edinburgh: Churchill Livingstone.

Roper, N., Logan, W. and Tierney, A. 1983. *Using a Model for Nursing.* Edinburgh: Churchill Livingstone.

Rose, A.M. 1980. A systematic summary of symbolic interaction theory. In Riehl and Roy 1980.

Schrock, R. A. 1981. Philosophical issues. In Hockey 1981.

Torres, G. 1985. The place of concepts and theories. In George 1985.

Walsh, M. 1989. Model example. In *Nursing Standard,* Issue 22, Vol. 3.

Chapter 2

Colledge, M. M. and Jones, D. (eds) 1979. *Readings in Nursing.* Edinburgh: Churchill Livingstone.

Henderson, V. 1969. *Basic Principles of Nursing Care.* New York: Macmillan.

Maslow, A. H. 1954. *Motivation and Personality.* New York: Harper & Row.

Roper, N. 1973. *Principles of Nursing.* Edinburgh: Churchill Livingstone.

Roper, N. 1976. *Clinical Experience in Nurse Education.* Edinburgh: Churchill Livingstone.

Roper, N. 1979. Nursing based on a model for living. In Colledge and Jones 1979.

Roper, N., Logan, W. and Tierney, A. 1985. *The Elements of Nursing,* 2nd. edn. Edinburgh: Churchill Livingstone.

Chapter 3

Bee, H. L. and Mitchell, S. K. 1980. *The Developing Person: a life span approach.* New York: Harper & Row.

Binnie, A., Bond, S., *et al.* 1984. *A Systematic Approach to Nursing Care.* Milton Keynes: Open University Press.

Bond, S. 1984. *A Systematic Approach to Nursing Care.* Cambridge: Open University.

Chapman, C. 1982. *Sociology for Nurses.* London: Bailliere Tindall.

Colledge, M. M. and Jones, D. (eds) 1979. *Readings in Nursing.* Edinburgh: Churchill Livingstone.

Erikson, E. H. 1950. *Childhood and Society,* 1st edn. New York: Norton.

McFarlane, J. 1980. Essays on nursing. (Project papers based on working papers of the Royal Commission on NHS, No. RC2.) London: Kings Fund Centre. (Cited in Binnie *et al.* 1984.)

Roper, N. 1979. Nursing based on a model for living. In Colledge and Jones 1979.

Roper, N., Logan, W. and Tierney, A. 1983. *Using a Model for Nursing.* Edinburgh: Churchill Livingstone.

Roper, N., Logan, W. and Tierney, A. 1985. *The Elements of Nursing*, 2nd edn. Edinburgh: Churchill Livingstone.

Stuart, G. 1953. *The Private World of Pain.* London: George Allen & Unwin. (Quoted in Chapman 1982.)

Wilson Barnett, J. 1978. Factors influencing patients' emotional reaction to hospitalisation. In *Journal of Advanced Nursing,* **3**.

Chapter 4

ABPI 1988. *Data Sheet Compendium.* London: Datapharm.

Ainslie, S. 1981. Sexuality and the cancer sufferer. In *Nursing Mirror,* **159** (10).

Boore, J. 1978. *Prescription for Recovery.* London: Royal College of Nursing.

Chapman, C. 1982. *Sociology for Nurses.* London: Bailliere Tindall.

David, J. 1988. Treatment Regimes. Unpublished lecture given at the Royal Hampshire County Hospital, Winchester, 16 May 1988.

Golden, J. 1980. Special aspects in surgery. In *Advanced Psychosomatic Medicine,* **10**.

Gooch, J. 1984. *The Other Side of Surgery.* London: Macmillan.

Hamilton-Smith, M. 1988. *The Importance of Nutrition.* Unpublished lecture given at the Royal Hampshire County Hospital, Winchester, May 1988.

Hamilton-Smith, S. 1972. *Nil by Mouth.* London: Royal College of Nursing.

Hayward, J. 1978. *Information: a prescription against pain.* London: Royal College of Nursing.

Hilgarde, E., Atkinson, R. and Atkinson, R. 1979. *Introduction to Psychology*, 7th edn. New York: Harcourt Brace Jovanovitch.

Illingworth, C. 1970. Post-operative thrombosis and pulmonary embolism. In *Nursing Times,* **66**(15).

Janis, I. 1983. *Short-Term Counselling.* New York: Yale University Press.

McCaffery, M. 1983. *Nursing the Patient in Pain.* London: Harper & Row. (Quoted in Roper *et al.* 1985.)

Parsons, T. 1966. On becoming a patient. In Folta, J. R., and Deck, F. (eds): *A Sociological Framework for Patient Care.* New York: Wiley.

Peters, D. 1983. Bowel preparation for surgery. In *Nursing Times,* **79**(28).

Rogers, C. 1951. *Client-Centred Therapy.* London: Houghton Mifflin.

Roper, N. 1976. *Clinical Experience in Nurse Education.* Edinburgh: Churchill Livingstone.

Roper, N., Logan, W. and Tierney, A. 1983. *Using a Model for Nursing.* Edinburgh: Churchill Livingstone.

Roper, N., Logan, W. and Tierney, A. 1985. *The Elements of Nursing*, 2nd edn. Edinburgh: Churchill Livingstone.

Selye, H. 1976. *Stress in Health and Disease.* London: Butterworth.
Suchman, E. A. 1965. Stages of illness and medical care. In *Journal of Health and Human Behaviour,* 5. (Quoted in Chapman 1982.)
Tortora, C. and Anagnostakos, N. 1981. *Principles of Anatomy and Physiology.* New York: Harper & Row.
Watson, P. G. 1983. The effects of short-term post-operative counselling on cancer/ostomy patients. In *Cancer Nursing,* Feb. 1983.
Wilson Barnett, J. 1978a. Factors affecting patients' emotional reaction to hospitalisation. In *Journal of Advanced Nursing,* 3.
Wilson Barnett, J. 1978b. In hospital: patients' feelings and opinions. In *Nursing Times Occasional paper,* 74(8), March 16th.
Woods, N. and Mandetta, A. 1975. Human sexuality in health and illness. In *Nursing Research,* 25.

Chapter 5

Binnie, A., Bond, S., *et al.* 1984. *A Systematic Approach to Nursing Care.* Milton Keynes: Open University Press.
Burr, M. L., Fainly, A. M. and Gilbert, J. F. 1989. Effects of change in fat, fish and fibre intakes on death and myocardial infarction. In *Lancet,* 2(8666).
Hannah, D. and Alimo, A. 1989. A heartwarming scheme. In *Nursing Times,* 85(11).
Hilgarde, E., Atkinson, R. and Atkinson, R. 1979. *Introduction to Psychology.* New York: Harcourt Brace Jovanovitch.
Kratz, C. R. 1979. *The Nursing Process.* London: Bailliere Tindall.
Long, B. C. and Phipps, W. J. 1985. *Essentials of Medical-Surgical Nursing: a nursing process approach.* St. Louis: Mosby.
McFarlane, J. 1980. Essays on nursing. (Project papers based on working papers of the Royal Commission on NHS, No. RC2). London: Kings Fund Centre. (Cited in Binnie *et al.* 1984.)
National Audit Office 1989. *National Health Service: coronary heart disease.* London: HMSO.
Norton, D., McLaren, R. and Exton-Smith, A. 1962. *An Investigation of Geriatric Nursing Problems in Hospital.* Edinburgh: Churchill Livingstone.
Roper, N., Logan, W. and Tierney, A. 1985. *The Elements of Nursing,* 2nd edn. Edinburgh: Churchill Livingstone.
Thompson, D. R. and Cordle, C. J. 1988. Support of wives of myocardial infarction patients. In *Journal of Advanced Nursing,* 13.
Tortora, G. and Anagnostakos, N. 1981. *Principles of Anatomy and Physiology.* New York: Harper & Row.
Wilson Barnett, J. 1988. Patient teaching or patient counselling. In *Journal of Advanced Nursing,* 13.

Chapter 6

Bee, H. and Mitchell, S. *The Developing Child*, 5th edn. New York: Harper & Row.

Bowlby, J. 1973. *Attachment and Loss: (2) Separation, anxiety and anger*. New York: Basic Books.

Coulson, D. 1988. A proper place for parents. In *Nursing Times*, **84**(19).

Dewar, A. and Glasper, A. 1987. Help hazard. In *Nursing Times*, **83**(51).

Erikson, E. H. 1950. *Childhood and Society*, 1st edn. New York: Norton.

Hawthorn, P. J. 1974. *Nurse – I Want my Mummy*. London: Royal College of Nursing.

HMSO 1959. *Report on the Welfare of Children in Hospital* (Chairman: H. Platt). London: HMSO.

Lewer, H. and Robertson, L. 1983. *Care of the Child*. London: Macmillan.

Roper, N., Logan, W. and Tierney, A. 1985. *The Elements of Nursing*, 2nd edn. Edinburgh: Churchill Livingstone.

Sadler, C. 1988. Being there. In *Nursing Times*, **84**(34).

Chapter 7

Closs, S. J., MacDonald, I. A. and Hawthorn, P. J. 1986. Factors affecting peri-operative body temperature. In *Journal of Advanced Nursing*, **11**(6).

Long, B. C. and Phipps, W. J. 1985. *Essentials of Medical-Surgical Nursing: a nursing process approach*. St. Louis: Mosby.

Lowthian, P. 1979. Turning clock system to prevent pressure sores. In *Nursing Mirror*, **148**.

Norton, D., McLaren, R. and Exton Smith, A. 1962. *An Investigation of Geriatric Nursing Problems in Hospital*. Edinburgh: Churchill Livingstone.

Roberts, A. 1989. Systems of life, No. 168: Senior systems (33). In *Nursing Times*, **85**(6).

Summerskill, H. 1976. Measurements of gastric function during digestion of ordinary solid meals in man. In *Gastroenterology*, **83**, 46–7. (Quoted in Walsh and Ford 1989.)

Thomlinson, D. 1987. To clean or not to clean? In *Nursing Times*, **83**.

Walsh, M. and Ford, P. 1989. We've always done it this way. In *Nursing Times*, **85**(41).

Chapter 8

Janis, I. 1983. *Short-Term Counselling*. New York: Yale University Press.

Long, B. C. and Phipps, W. J. 1985. *Essentials of Medical-Surgical Nursing: a nursing process approach*. St. Louis: Mosby.

Manning, V. 1989. No more watching the clock. In *Nursing Times*, **85**(26).

Maslow, A. J. 1954. *Motivation and Personality*. New York: Harper & Row.

Tortora, G. and Anagnostakos, N. 1981. *Principles of Anatomy and Physiology*. New York: Harper & Row.

Wilson Barnett, J. 1988. Patient teaching or patient counselling. In *Journal of Advanced Nursing*, **13**.

Chapter 9

Aggleton, P. and Chalmers, H. 1987. Models of nursing, nursing practice and nurse education. In *Journal of Advanced Nursing*, **12**.

Binnie, A., Bond, S. *et al.* 1984. *A Systematic Approach to Nursing Care*. Milton Keynes: Open University Press.

Botha, M.E. 1989. Theory development in perspective: the role of conceptual frameworks and models in theory development. In *Journal of Advanced Nursing*, **14**.

Cassons, J. 1980. *Dying – the greatest adventure of my life*. London: Christian Medical Fellowship.

Clark, D. 1988. Framework for care. In *Nursing Times*, **84**(35).

Clark, J. 1986. A model for health visiting. In Kershaw and Salvage 1986.

Clark, J. and Bishop, J. 1988. Model-making. In *Nursing Times*, **84**(27).

Colledge, M. M. and Jones, D. (eds) 1979. *Readings in Nursing*. Edinburgh: Churchill Livingstone.

Donaldson, S. K. and Crowley, D. M. 1978. The discipline of nursing. In *Nursing Outlook*, **26**. (Quoted in Fawcett 1989.)

Erikson, E. H. 1950. *Childhood and Society*, 1st edn. New York: Norton.

Farmer, E. 1986. Exploring the issues. In Kershaw and Salvage 1986.

Fawcett, J. 1989. *Analysis and Evaluation of Conceptual Models of Nursing*, 2nd edn. Philadelphia: Davis.

Flaskerud, J. H. and Halloran, E.J. 1980. Areas of agreement in nursing theory development. In *Advances in Nursing Science*, **3**(1).

Hanucharurnkul, S. 1989. Comparative analysis of Orem's and King's theories. In *Journal of Advanced Nursing*, **14**.

Henderson, V. 1969. *Basic Principles of Nursing Care*. New York: Macmillan.

Jackson, M. 1986. On maps and models. In *Senior Nurse*, **15**(4).

Jourard, S. M. 1964. *The Transparent Self*. New York: Van Nostrand. (Quoted in Roper 1976.)

Kershaw, B. and Salvage, J. (eds) 1986. *Models for Nursing*. Chichester: Wiley.

Kubler-Ross, E. 1969. *On Death and Dying*. New York: Macmillan.

Lewis, T. 1988. Leaping the chasm between nursing theory and practice. In *Journal of Advanced Nursing*, **13**, 345–51.

McFarlane, J. 1980. *Essays on Nursing*. (Project papers based on working papers of the Royal Commission of NHS, No. RC2.) London: Kings Fund Centre. (Cited in Binnie *et al.* 1984.)

Maslow, A. H. 1954. *Motivation and Personality*. New York: Harper & Row.

Meleis, A. I. 1985. *Theoretical Nursing: development and practice*. Pennsylvania, USA: Lippincott.

Minshull, J., Ross, K. and Turner, J. 1986. The human-needs model of nursing. In *Journal of Advanced Nursing*, **11**, 643–9.

Office of Health Economics, 1971. *Prospects in health*. London: OHE. (Quoted in Roper *et al.* 1985.)

Pearson, A. 1983. *The Clinical Nursing Unit*. London: Heinemann Medical Books.

Roper, N. 1976. *Clinical Experience in Nurse Education*. Edinburgh: Churchill Livingstone.

Roper, N. 1979. Nursing based on a model for living. In Colledge and Jones 1979.

Roper, N., Logan, W. and Tierney, A. 1980. *The Elements of Nursing*. Edinburgh: Churchill Livingstone.

Roper, N., Logan, W. and Tierney, A. 1981. *Learning to Use the Process of Nursing*. Edinburgh: Churchill Livingstone.

Roper, N., Logan, W. and Tierney, A. 1983a. Problems or needs? In *Nursing Mirror*, June 8th.

Roper, N., Logan, W. and Tierney, A. 1983b. *Using a Model for Nursing*. Edinburgh: Churchill Livingstone.

Roper, N., Logan, W. and Tierney, A. 1985. *The Elements of Nursing*. Edinburgh: Churchill Livingstone.

Schwartz, D., Henley, B. and Zeitz, L. 1964. *The Elderly Ambulant Patient*. New York: Macmillan. (Quoted in Roper 1976.)

Thibodeau, J. A. 1983. *Nursing Models: analysis and evaluation*. Monterey, CA: Wadsworth.

Tierney, A. 1984. The first step of the nursing process. In Binnie *et al.* 1984.

Tyler, R. W. 1952. Distinctive attributes of education for the professions. In *Social Work Journal*, **33**. (Quoted in Roper 1976.)

Walker, L. O. and Nicholson, R. 1980. Criteria for evaluating nursing process models. In *Nurse Educator*, 5(5). (Quoted in Fawcett 1989.)

Wilding, C., Wells, M. and Wilson, J. 1988. A model for family care. In *Nursing Times*, **84**(15), 38–41.

Wilson, J. 1972. *Philosophy and Educational Research*. Windsor: National Foundation for Educational Research in England and Wales. (Quoted in Roper 1976.)

Wright, S. G. 1986. *Building and Using a Model of Nursing*. London: Edward Arnold.